The STATIN DISASTER

David Brownstein, M.D.

For further copies of *The Statin Disaster*:
Call: 1-888-647-5616 or send a check or money order in the amount of:
$23.00 ($18.00 plus $5.00 shipping and handling) or for Michigan residents $24.08 ($18.00 plus $5.00 shipping and handling, plus $1.08 sales tax) to:

> Medical Alternatives Press
> 4173 Fieldbrook
> West Bloomfield, Michigan 48323

The Statin Disaster
Copyright © 2015 by David Brownstein, M.D.
All Rights Reserved
No part of this book may be reproduced without written consent from the publisher.

ISBN: 978-0-9840869-3-1
Medical Alternatives Press
4173 Fieldbrook
West Bloomfield, Michigan 48323
(248) 851-3372
(888) 647-5616
www.drbrownstein.com

Acknowledgements

I gratefully acknowledge the help I have received from my friends and colleagues in putting this book together. This book could not have been published without help from the editors—my wife Allison, Dr. Ira Goodman, Dawn Malott, Angela Biggs, and Janet Darnell.

I would also like to thank my patients. It is your search for safe and effective natural treatments that is the driving force behind holistic medicine. You have accompanied me down this path and I appreciate each and every one of you.

And, to my staff. Thank you so very much for taking this trip with me. Without your help and support, none of this would be possible. I do appreciate all of your hard work and your dedication.

A Word of Caution to the Reader

The information presented in this book is based on the training and professional experience of the author. The treatments recommended in this book should not be undertaken without first consulting a physician. Proper laboratory and clinical monitoring is essential to achieving the goals of finding safe and natural treatments. This book was written for informational and educational purposes only. It is not intended to be used as medical advice.

ABOUT THE AUTHOR

David Brownstein, M.D. is a Board-Certified family physician who utilizes the best of conventional and alternative therapies. He is the Medical Director for the Center for Holistic Medicine in West Bloomfield, MI. He is a graduate of the University of Michigan and Wayne State University School of Medicine. Dr. Brownstein is a member of the American Academy of Family Physicians and the International College of Integrative Medicine (ICIM). He is the father of two beautiful girls, Hailey and Jessica and is a retired soccer coach. Dr. Brownstein has lectured internationally about his success using natural items. Dr. Brownstein has authored thirteen books: *Iodine: Why You Need It, Why You Can't Live Without It, 5th Edition; Vitamin B12 for Health; Drugs That Don't Work and Natural Therapies That Do, 2nd Edition; The Miracle of Natural Hormones, 3rd Edition; Overcoming Thyroid Disorders 3rd Edition; Overcoming Arthritis; Salt Your Way to Health, 2nd Edition; The Guide To Healthy Eating, 2nd Edition; The Guide to a Gluten-Free Diet, 2nd Edition; The Guide to a Dairy-Free Diet; The Soy Deception; The Skinny on Fats* and *The Statin Disaster.*

Dr. Brownstein's office is located at:

Center for Holistic Medicine
5821 W. Maple Rd.
Ste. 192
West Bloomfield, MI 48322
248.851.1600
www.centerforholisticmedicine.com

CONTENTS

	Foreword	7
	Preface	9
Chapter 1:	My Story	15
Chapter 2:	Statins, Statins, and More Statins	21
Chapter 3:	What is Cholesterol, HDL, and LDL?	31
Chapter 4:	Cholesterol: What Is It Good For?	51
Chapter 5:	The Cholesterol = Heart Disease Hypothesis	67
Chapter 6:	The Biosynthetic Pathway for Cholesterol	85
Chapter 7:	Statistics, Damn Statistics, and Statins	101
Chapter 8:	Cholesterol Guidelines: Nonsense Best Avoided	133
Chapter 9:	Adverse Effects of Statins	155
Chapter 10:	Women and Statins	191
Chapter 11:	Cholesterol and Hormones	205
Chapter 12:	Cholesterol and Hypothyroidism	227
Chapter 13:	Cholesterol and Iodine	247
Chapter 14:	Diet and Heart Disease	261
Chapter 15:	Final Thoughts	281
	Appendix	294
	Index	295

DEDICATION

To Allison, my best friend and wife. I could not do any of this without you.

To physicians who are not satisfied with the dogma and who are willing to search for a new paradigm that promotes health.

To my staff: Thanks so much for all of your help and encouragement. I appreciate all of your hard work.

And, to my patients. Thank you for being interested in what I am interested in.

Last, but certainly not least. I dedicate this book to my friend John. Thank you for that special place to write.

FOREWORD

As you read this book, over 1000 lawsuits have been filed against Pfizer claiming that Lipitor caused diabetes. But that's only one of more than two dozen serious adverse reactions associated with statin medications. Hopefully, the tide is changing and that awareness of statin injury and lack of benefit is rising among the public and federal regulators.

If so, Dr. Brownstein's book, *The Statin Disaster*, comes at an auspicious time when a sentinel work like this can permeate public knowledge and escalate legal challenges against this world health scourge. Almost ten years of FDA data reveal the staggering extent of serious reactions associated with statins. Dr. Brownstein has faithfully disclosed those statistics that continue to multiply due to the almost universal recommendations of statin use. I have witnessed hundreds of tragic stories of statin injuries including those among our veterans who survived war only to be damaged by misguided and unnecessary cholesterol therapy drugs.

In *The Statin Disaster*, Dr. Brownstein provides us with an accurate and revealing perspective of the true nature of statin drugs. Using his usual clarity and straightforward style, Dr. Brownstein delivers the clinical support and evidence to help all readers understand the dangers and distortions of statin therapy even while they are being heavily promoted in some medical offices. Armed with this resource, patients will be able to defend themselves against bullying by misguided healthcare providers and Big Pharma.

Philip Blair, M.D.

Colonel, Medical Corps, U.S. Army (retired)
CEO of AbleDoc, Inc, Disease Management Services
Chief Medical Officer, Pro Health Advisor
Member of THINCS: The International Network of Cholesterol Skeptics

PREFACE

It has always amazed me how the pharmaceutical industrial complex has managed to convince the overwhelming majority of the public, as well as most physicians, that statins play a vital role in prevention and treatment of cardiovascular disease. It is a modern wonder of marketing and public relations that they have succeeded in doing this in spite of the cold hard evidence, much of which they produced.

Their best evidence for statin drugs shows only an absolute benefit of 1-2% over three years for most cohorts. In other words, the patient is not helped 98-99% of the time but is significantly disadvantaged as well. Dr. Brownstein's thoughtful analysis will explore this key point. Yes statins lower cholesterol and lower LDL-cholesterol as well as work to lower C-reactive protein (CRP) quite nicely. The only problem is that they do not significantly lower cardiovascular events or death rate.

Imagine if you were in Las Vegas at a roulette wheel that had 98 red slots and 2 black ones. I would bet on the red every time but somehow Big Pharma has convinced us that black is the right bet.

I would like to know how Big Pharma pulls this off and convinces everyone that statins are beneficial. Is it the carefully selected and meticulously groomed "thought leaders" who are paid handsomely to show the slides and put their names on the articles that have been created for them? Or is it the total control of medical education from first year medical school to all levels of post-graduate training? How about the influence they exert over the medical journals via advertising dollars? Or maybe it's the statisticians? I wish we could bottle up this astounding marketing ability and apply it to something worthwhile.

Drugs used to be discovered, now they are marketed and sold. In 2010 Pfizer set a new standard by topping $50 billion (yes that's 50 billion) in sales. In 2015, it is estimated that the global sales of pharmaceuticals will approach $1 trillion (yes that's 1 trillion).

Think about these facts:

- In 2005, Americans spent $250 billion on pharmaceuticals – more than the entire Gross Domestic Product (GDP) of Argentina and Peru.
- In 2004, Americans spent more on pharmaceuticals than on gasoline or fast food.
- Americans spend twice as much on pharmaceuticals than on higher education or automobiles.
- Americans spend more on pharmaceuticals than Japan, Germany, France, Italy, Spain, UK, Australia, New Zealand, Canada, Mexico, Brazil, and Argentina COMBINED.
- 65% of our entire population takes pharmaceuticals, and the elderly take on average 30 prescriptions/year.

- Pharmaceuticals kill more people than diabetes or Alzheimer's disease.
- There are over 100,000 U.S. pharmaceutical sales reps - about one for every six physicians.
- Between 1998 and 2004, the U.S. pharmaceutical industry spent more on lobbying than any other industry.
- Only the USA and New Zealand allow direct-to-consumer pharmaceutical advertising.
- 10- 25% of pharmaceutical revenue is spent on promotion.

Dr. Brownstein will explore Big Pharma's sleight of hand with statistics and he will point out that most (greater than 95%) physicians do not understand this. The sleight of hand is successful because of the innumeracy of most physicians. We all know what illiteracy is, innumeracy is the same concept applied to numbers. As Mark Twain once said: "A person who won't read has no advantage over one who can't read". Simply put, most physicians do not understand how to read and correctly interpret the statistics in medical journal articles. They do not understand relative risk, absolute risk, number-needed-to-treat (NNT), number-needed-to-harm (NNH), or odds ratios. I do understand these concepts, have written about them and can explain them. However, when faced with my own cardiologist, armed with my own lab report showing an elevated surrogate marker (cholesterol level), telling me I need to take a statin, I became like a deer in the headlights and blindly acceded to his wishes! I later developed adverse effects. I came to my senses, and stopped the drug. Why should I sacrifice my well-being now for a one percent chance that I might avoid a cardiac event in the next ten years? This time, I am betting on red.

There are two main reasons why statins have been widely used and neither one has anything to do with rational scientific evidence. The first reason is that prescribing these medications is now considered "the standard of care". In other words, everyone does it. The other reason is that these decisions are based on fear in the context of emotional arousal. When your white-coated cardiologist/internist/ family doctor looks you in the eye and says you need this drug it is usually the end of the story. All thought stops, and the limbic system (the center of emotion) takes over. Your frontal lobe should be functioning but it is not. A layman has almost no defense against the "full court press" they face by the nurse, physician, abnormal lab reports, and all their friends who are on statins. Why would intelligent physicians continue to do this? There are only two reasons: either they do not know better or they do know better but just go along with the herd. Sorry if I am not politically correct, but these are the facts.

Unfortunately, this is the story of the way medicine is practiced much of the time: something sounds like a good idea and it becomes the standard-of-care. Opposing evidence is ignored and independent thinking is left at the door of the thought leaders. This is especially true for procedures since they are not regulated by the FDA. Drugs undergo rigorous trials but clinical significance is conflated with statistical significance which harms people. It's pathetic.

I have known Dr. David Brownstein for many years. He is remarkable in his fresh, unbiased approach to many subjects and this includes his thoughtful approach to statins. He is not in anyone's pocket, reads the underlying literature, and comes to his own conclusions. This alone sets him apart from the crowd. People have asked me how he does so much: a busy practice with enormous experience in IV therapies, thyroid and iodine treatment, his blog, newsletters, multiple books, and lecture schedule. His practice is full. Think about what that means. Other physicians are busy attending marketing seminars, spending money on advertising, and promoting themselves in any way possible. David does none of that since patients are banging down the doors. Why? He is honest, rational, and he has only the patient's best interest in mind, and everyone can see it.

I am sure the reader will remember the tale of the *Wizard of Oz*. Dorothy looked behind the curtain to expose the wizard. Dr. Brownstein will look behind the curtain in *The Statin Disaster* to expose the wizards of Big Pharma. These wizards, however, do not use loudspeakers, smoke billows, and mechanical devices.

Instead, they use thought leaders, statistical confusion, and monetary influence to succeed in pulling off one of the most incredible deceptions mankind has ever seen. Dr. Brownstein will show you the emperor has no clothes and the wizard is blowing smoke. This is an important book that I hope you read carefully. It could save your life.

Ira L Goodman, MD FACS, ABIHM, FAARM, ABAARM

Chapter 1

My Story

CHAPTER 1: MY STORY

I graduated from medical school in 1989 and finished my residency three years later. When I started practicing medicine, I began as I was trained. I was trained to make a diagnosis and then prescribe the drug to treat that diagnosis. Nowhere in my training was I taught about what health is and how to maintain it.

At the beginning of my career, I bought into all I was taught in medical school. I thought drugs could treat everything. However, the actual practice of medicine changed things. I quickly began to see that nearly all the drugs I was trained to prescribe did not treat the underlying cause of any illness; rather they treated the symptoms of the illness.

It took me six months of practicing conventional medicine before I began to feel uneasy. After successfully treating my father's heart condition with bioidentical, natural hormones, I knew that this was the type of medicine I wanted to practice. (His story is discussed in more detail in Chapter 11.) From that moment on, I found my passion; studying and applying natural therapies to treat the underlying cause of my patients' illnesses.

My dad's case was very interesting. His cholesterol level fell over 100mg/dl without changing his diet or habits. Since I saw the positive changes in my father's health, I began to study what could be the underlying cause of heart disease. I felt that only by understanding the underlying cause could I formulate an effective treatment plan.

Many of my heart disease patients suffer from hormonal imbalances, particularly thyroid hormone imbalances. When I studied the literature on hypothyroidism and heart disease, I was stunned to see that there was well over 100 years of literature detailing how and why an underactive thyroid gland can cause an elevated cholesterol level. I was not taught that in my medical training. I was taught that elevated cholesterol caused heart disease.

When I started evaluating my heart disease patients for thyroid and other hormonal and nutritional problems, I began to see a pattern. Many of them were suffering with an underactive thyroid. Their elevated cholesterol level was just the symptom of the underlying problem—hypothyroidism. In these cases, why would I treat the symptom—elevated cholesterol levels—instead of the underlying problem—hypothyroidism?

I began to look with skepticism on the whole 'cholesterol is responsible for causing heart disease' theory. In this book, I refer to this as the "cholesterol = heart disease hypothesis". My skepticism lead me to research statin drugs.

When I began my research of statin drugs, I started with looking at their biochemical effects in the body. Once I learned how they worked–they poisoned a crucial enzyme (HMG CoA reductase) in the body—I knew that the data behind the positive studies must have been manipulated. How could this class of drugs have such positive benefits when the drugs poison a crucial enzyme? They can't. And, they don't.

I wrote this book to provide the reader with the knowledge he/she will need to make an informed decision about whether to take a statin drug or not. This information is not readily available as most health care professionals do not understand how to properly evaluate a research article's statistics.

Statin drugs are minimally (1-3%) effective at preventing heart attacks and death. That means they are 97-99% ineffective for those who take them. Their side effect profile alone should push the FDA to withdraw them and should also give pause to any patient taking them.

This book will also provide you with answers on how to avoid becoming a heart patient.

One last note. I belong to an online group called THINCS—The International Network of Cholesterol Skeptics (www.thincs.org). This group consists of 103 of the most intelligent doctors, nutritionists, engineers, and PhD's, (if I forgot anyone, I apologize) that I have ever had the privilege to share information and ideas with. The group was started by our leader, Uffe Ravnskov, M.D.

I have learned much from my friends and colleagues in this online group and would like to personally thank everyone in this group for sharing their thoughts and ideas. I would encourage the reader to go to www.thincs.org for more information about this group.

Chapter 2

Statins, Statins, and More Statins

CHAPTER 2: INTRODUCTION

No one would fault you if you think statins should be put into the water supply. They are touted as miracle drugs that help us reduce our risk of heart disease.

Statins are the most profitable medications in the history of Big Pharma. From 2003 to 2012, the percentage of adults aged 40 and over using a statin increased from 20% to 28%.[1] Currently, over 25 million Americans take a daily statin medication.[2] In 2011, over $4.4 billion was spent for the statin medication Crestor® while another $7.7 billion was spent for Lipitor®. If we adopt the new (2013) cholesterol-lowering guidelines (discussed in Chapter 8), 56 million American adults between the ages of 40-75 would be eligible to take a statin medication.

I guess the United States of America must be suffering from a statin-deficiency syndrome. (That last sentence was stated with sarcasm).

Is everything so rosy with statins? I say the answer is easy, "No!"

DOES CHOLESTEROL CAUSE HEART DISEASE?

For over 100 years, conventional medicine has been fixated on the idea that cholesterol is responsible for causing the epidemic of heart disease. In fact, The Powers-That-Be and most conventional health care providers are convinced that cholesterol is the root cause of heart disease. The "Powers-That-Be" include the American Heart Association, the American Medical Association, the American College of Cardiology, the Food and Drug Administration, and nearly every other mainstream medical organization.

Figuring out what causes heart attacks is big business as heart disease has been our number one killer for over 60 years. Conventional medicine has an easy-to-understand approach to this problem. It starts with cholesterol that blocks the coronary arteries causing a heart attack. Therefore, they believe that we must lower our cholesterol levels to the lowest possible number. Of course, this can only occur with cholesterol-lowering medications.

EVIDENCE-BASED MEDICINE AND STATINS

The Powers-That-Be love to use the term "evidence-based

medicine" (EBM) when they write about statin medications. They cite study after study showing the heart benefits of lowering cholesterol via statin use. And, they claim that statins have very few adverse effects.

I see nothing wrong with evidence-based medicine. Health care providers should use the best evidence at hand to make an informed decision about which therapy would be most beneficial for the patient in front of them. However, there has never been a controlled study which proves that EBM results in better outcomes than treating by clinical experience. It's a starting point, nothing more.

Furthermore, I think most health care providers are not making evidence-based decisions because they do not understand how to comprehend medical research articles. This is particularly true about statin research.

WHY HEALTH CARE PROVIDERS CAN'T EVALUATE THE STUDIES

For physicians, the problem starts in medical school. There is so much information thrown at aspiring doctors that they just try to survive. No one teaches them how to properly read a medical journal article and understand how the authors came to the conclusion that they did. I should know, because I was one of them.

To properly read research articles, one has to have a good understanding of statistics. I have been teaching medical students and residents for over 20 years. Over this time period, I have seen hundreds of students rotate through my office. At the first visit I always hand the student a research article and tell them to summarize the results and tell me if the therapy was effective in the population that was treated.

Over the years, only one student was able to dissect the article and point out that the therapy studied was not very effective even though the abstract for the article claimed the therapy was 50% effective.

The reason the medical students and residents as well as most health care providers cannot understand how to evaluate a research article is that they do not understand statistics. I teach them how to look past the statistical analyses used in nearly all medical research so that they can decide whether the therapy was useful or not. Chapter 7 will review this topic in more detail. Finally, it is important to keep in mind that statistical significance is not the same as clinical significance.

STATINS: HELPFUL FOR PREVENTING HEART DISEASE?

That is the key question and the purpose of writing this

book. I will show you that the benefits of statins in preventing and/or treating heart disease is far outweighed by the harm that they cause.

Statins are prescribed either to prevent heart disease or to treat it. If someone has never had a history of heart disease and they are prescribed a statin, it would be prescribed for primary prevention—in an attempt to prevent heart disease or a heart attack. If a patient already has heart disease or has suffered a heart attack in the past, they would be prescribed a statin medication for secondary prevention—in order to try to prevent another heart-related problem.

It is important to keep the nomenclature clear when discussing statin use. I will use the term primary and secondary prevention throughout this book.

The benefits of statins are miniscule with both primary and secondary prevention. There are zero studies showing any significant benefits with using statins for primary prevention. For secondary prevention, the best of the statin studies have shown only a 1-3.5% reduction in heart attacks from using statin medications. That means, for secondary prevention, the drugs failed for 96.5-99% of those who took them. And, keep in mind, these same patients were exposed to the potential for adverse effects from statins which include: neurological, musculoskeletal, and cardiovascular problems as well as increasing the risk for diabetes. And, I am not even bringing up the idea of how much it costs to treat so few—but I will.

STATINS AND STATISTICS

Chapter 7 discusses how Big Pharma manipulates statistics to show an enhanced effectiveness of statin medications. In that chapter, I will show you the difference between relative and absolute risk in regards to statin therapy. Throughout this book, I have quoted many studies related to statins. I will point out the absolute risk reduction (AR) and the relative risk reduction (RR) when a study is analyzed.

FINAL THOUGHTS

Statin drugs have been prescribed for nearly 20 years. You would think that we would see marked declines in heart disease rates if they were truly the wonder drugs that The Big Pharma Cartel claims they are. I can assure you they are not.

Statins are the biggest fraud in modern medicine. They have been found to work in a very small percentage of those who take them. That might be okay if statins had no adverse effects and were relatively inexpensive. However, statins are associated with severe adverse effects. And, statins are not cheap. When you factor in the idea that they are the most profitable medications in the history of Big Pharma, the cost is almost unimaginable.

I will show you the fallacy of the idea that cholesterol is responsible for causing the heart disease epidemic. Cholesterol is an essential substance that we cannot live without.

Statins are too expensive and dangerous. Furthermore, they help very few patients. I believe that statins should be pulled from the marketplace.

[1] NHANES. Data Briefs. N. 177. Dec. 2014
[2] CBS News. Accessed 1.27.15 from: http://www.cbsnews.com/news/13-million-more-americans-would-take-statins-if-new-guidelines-followed-study/

Chapter 3

What Is Cholesterol, HDL, and LDL?

CHAPTER 3: INTRODUCTION

Cholesterol is a waxy, fat-like substance that is produced in the body and obtained from the diet. Every cell needs and requires cholesterol for optimal functioning. It is an essential component of every cell membrane. In fact, cholesterol is a precursor substrate for vitamin D, our sex hormones like estrogen and testosterone, and is vital for brain function. The chemical structure of cholesterol is shown in Figure 1.

This chapter will review the common terminology of different molecules associated with cholesterol transport such as high density lipoprotein (HDL) and low density lipoprotein (LDL). I know this material can be boring to some, but it is important to understand how and why cholesterol is transported throughout the body. Statins disrupt the normal production of cholesterol and cause many adverse effects. This chapter will show you that there is no such thing as "good" or "bad" cholesterol. Furthermore, I will help you understand why statins cause so many health issues and why statins do not have a positive effect on reducing heart disease for the vast majority of individuals who take them.

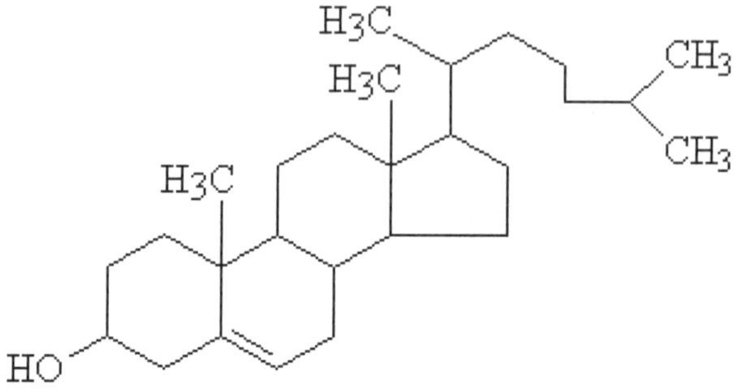

Figure 1: Structure of Cholesterol

"GOOD" AND "BAD" CHOLESTEROL?

The American Heart Association states, "There are two types of cholesterol: "good" and "bad." Too much of one type—or not enough of another—can put you at risk of coronary heart disease, heart attack, or stroke. It's important to know the levels of cholesterol in your blood so that you and your doctor can determine the best strategy to lower your risk."[1]

They make it sound so simple; just lower the "bad" cholesterol or raise the "good" cholesterol and everything will be fine. However, things are not that simple. In fact, this whole idea of "good" and "bad" cholesterol is wrong. Let me explain.

Cholesterol is produced in nearly all tissues of the body. The liver produces the most cholesterol—about 20% of the body's total production. The cholesterol production rate, which includes both endogenously synthesized and absorbed cholesterol, is approximately one gram per day. The average cholesterol intake is thought to be about 300mg/day with only about half of that amount actually being absorbed. Endogenous synthesis of cholesterol accounts for over two-thirds of the body's cholesterol level.[2] The human body is designed to tightly control cholesterol absorption and synthesis as well as its degradation.

For those who think cholesterol is an evil substance that we need to lower, I will pose the following question: If cholesterol is such a bad substance, then why is there such an intricate mechanism built into the body in order to produce and maintain adequate cholesterol levels?

WHAT IS CHOLESTEROL?

Cholesterol is an interesting substance. Many mistakenly refer to cholesterol as a fat. It is not. Notice (see Figure 1) the 'OH' molecule attached to the end of the cholesterol structure. (For the non-chemistry majors, it is illustrated as 'HO' in Figure 1). This indicates that cholesterol is an alcohol. It is not a fat molecule, but, like fats, it is also insoluble and does not dissolve in the bloodstream.

Since fats and cholesterol are needed by every cell, tissue, and organ of the body, the body has been designed with a perfect mechanism to transport fats and cholesterol throughout the body. These specialized transport mechanisms are known as lipoproteins.

LIPOPROTEINS: ESSENTIAL TRANSPORT MOLECULES

Lipoproteins can be considered to be like taxi cabs. These taxi cabs are designed to carry insoluble fat and cholesterol to the tissues and cells throughout the body. There are five major groups of lipoproteins:

- Chylomicrons

- VLDL (very-low-density lipoprotein)

- IDL (intermediate-density lipoprotein)

- LDL (low-density lipoprotein)

- HDL (high-density lipoprotein)

Chylomicrons are named from the Greek words 'chylo'—milky fluid—and micron—small size. They contain mostly triglycerides (about 90%) and also have a small amount of cholesterol (1-3%). They are produced in the intestines and are designed to carry fat, after a meal, from the intestines to the fat cells of various tissues in the body where the fat is utilized for energy or storage.

Triglycerides are a type of fat which is found in the blood. After a meal, the body will convert excess calories into triglycerides. Since fat is not soluble in the bloodstream, triglycerides are carried by lipoproteins. The triglycerides are deposited in the fat cells and can be broken down for energy when the body needs them.

VLDL particles are simply smaller-sizes of chylomicrons. They are produced in the intestines and the liver. VLDLs contain about 60% triglycerides and 10-15% cholesterol. As the VLDLs lose their triglycerides to the different tissues of the body, they become a smaller size and can now be referred to as intermediate-density lipoproteins or IDLPs. As IDLPs lose their triglycerides to the tissues, they become smaller and are now referred to as low density lipoproteins or LDLs. LDLs contain a higher content of cholesterol and lower triglyceride concentration as compared to VLDLs and the IDLPs

High density lipoprotein (HDL) is the smallest lipoprotein. Like the other lipoproteins, HDLs enable the transport of fat throughout the body. HDLs are produced in the liver. Their job is to gather excess or unused cholesterol from the tissues and return it to the liver. This pathway is sometimes referred to as the reverse cholesterol transport pathway. Once in the liver, bile salts (secreted from the gall bladder) help eliminate excess cholesterol from the body.

LDL and HDL are inappropriately referred to as "bad" and "good" cholesterol, respectively. LDLs and HDLs are not cholesterol molecules—they are lipoproteins. They carry fat and cholesterol throughout the body.

LOW-DENSITY LIPOPROTEINS

Since LDLs carry most of the cholesterol to the tissues of the body, the total cholesterol amount on the blood test will parallel LDL levels (referred to as LDL-cholesterol on laboratory tests). In other words, a higher total cholesterol will reflect with higher LDL-cholesterol laboratory results. Similarly, a lower total cholesterol level will have a lower LDL-cholesterol level on blood testing.

You would think that LDL is a terrible substance that we do not need in our bodies. However, nothing could be further from the truth. We cannot live without LDLs. Nearly all cardiologists are focused on lowering LDL levels through using medications—statins—which are associated with a host of severe adverse effects. However, they do not acknowledge (or do not understand) that LDLs have very important physiologic functions in the body.

As previously mentioned, when cells need cholesterol, the signal is sent to the LDLs to deliver more cholesterol. They carry cholesterol from the liver—where it is produced—to the tissues of the body. Approximately 70% of the cholesterol in the body is carried by LDLs.

PLEIOTROPIC EFFECTS OF LDL MOLECULES: ANTI-INFECTIVE PROPERTIES

LDLs have antimicrobial effects. In fact, LDLs have been shown to be effective at neutralizing bacterial toxins.[3] [4] Furthermore, LDLs have been shown to have positive effects at inhibiting Staphylococcus infection.[5]

Once you understand that LDLs have important antimicrobial attributes, it is not hard to predict what may occur when someone takes a drug that inhibits LDL production. Inhibiting LDLs could be predicted to cause problems with the immune system because it has lost part of its antimicrobial capabilities. In other words, the immune system, with poorly functioning LDLs or with a low concentration of LDLs, could be more susceptible to infection.

Animal studies have found that LDLs can bind and neutralize endotoxins from gram-negative bacteria.[6] Furthermore, studies have found that pre-incubation of the endotoxins with LDLs before injection into animals decreased the mortality of the animals.[7] Other studies have found that injection of lipoproteins markedly reduced the mortality in animals after endotoxin administration.[8] Mice who have low levels of LDLs are sensitive to the toxic effects of endotoxins.[9]

Studies have shown that young men with a previous sexually transmitted illness who also had low cholesterol, when compared to men with high cholesterol, had a two-fold increase in testing positive with human immunodeficiency virus (HIV).[10]

Researchers looked at the correlation between mortality and cholesterol levels.[11] They found an inverse correlation between cholesterol levels and mortality from gastrointestinal and respiratory illnesses. In other words, the lower the cholesterol levels, the higher the death rate from gastrointestinal and respiratory diseases. Keep in mind that a lowered cholesterol level means there will be a lowered LDL-cholesterol level on blood testing. That would explain why multiple studies have found an inverse correlation with cholesterol levels and mortality: lower cholesterol levels are associated with a higher mortality rate.[12,13]

Similar to LDLs, triglycerides also have anti-infective properties. Researchers showed that bacterial sepsis is associated with elevated triglyceride and other lipoprotein levels.[14] The authors state that lipoproteins can bind and neutralize bacterial endotoxin. Furthermore, they conclude that "...data demonstrating the capacity of {triglyceride-rich} lipoproteins to bind {bacterial endotoxin} protect against {bacterial endotoxin}-induced toxicity and modulate the overall host response to...bacterial toxin." In other words, the body produces more triglycerides and LDLs in order to help fight an infection.

In many illnesses, including heart disease, cholesterol and LDL levels are elevated. Often this is due to a long-standing infectious process. In this case, the elevated cholesterol and LDL-cholesterol levels are like the warning lights in your automobile. In the case of an infection, the elevated cholesterol and LDL-cholesterol blood levels are the warning lights signaling that there is an infectious problem occurring. The worst thing to do in this case is to prescribe a medication that would inhibit the production of either cholesterol or LDL as their antimicrobial effects will be lost.

NEW ANTI-LDL MEDICATIONS

One final thought on LDLs. There are new medications that Big Pharma is working on that block the LDL receptors. They are known as PCSK9 inhibitors. Yes, this new class of medications will lower LDL-cholesterol levels, but I predict their use will be associated with adverse effects including an increase in serious infections. I do not think PCSK9 will be an effective treatment for heart disease as it will disrupt a normal physiologic process in the body: the binding of LDL to its receptor. Since LDL cannot bind to its receptor, the body will lower the production of LDLs. As stated above, this decline of LDL production could be predicted to lead to an increase in infections and mortality.

HIGH-DENSITY LIPOPROTEINS

HDLs are produced in the liver. As previously mentioned, they are responsible for retrieving excess cholesterol molecules in the periphery and returning them to the liver.

HDLs are often referred to as the "good" cholesterol since they return excess and unused cholesterol to the liver. HDL-cholesterol is the term for the laboratory test of HDLs.

HDLs do not fluctuate as much as LDLs. In other words, there are genetic factors that control HDL levels to a greater degree when they are compared to LDLs. Many claim that elevated HDLs protect against heart disease.[15][16] However, there are other studies which fail to show a cardiac benefit of raising HDLs.[17]

It is unclear whether elevated HDLs may confer a protective effect in heart disease. Cholesteryl ester transfer protein inhibitors (CETP), niacin, and fibrates have all been shown to raise HDL-cholesterol levels. A meta-analysis or randomized controlled trials of these three classes of agents was performed in order to determine their effects on mortality and cardiovascular events.[18] A total of 39 trials, encompassing 117,411 subjects, were reviewed. The researchers reported, "Neither niacin, fibrates, nor CETP inhibitors, three highly effective agents for increasing high density lipoprotein levels, reduced all-cause mortality, coronary heart disease mortality, myocardial infarction, or stroke in patients treated with statins. Although observational studies might suggest a simplistic hypothesis for high density lipoprotein cholesterol, that increasing the levels pharmacologically would generally reduce cardiovascular events, in the current era of widespread use of statins in dyslipidaemia, substantial trials of these three agents do not support this concept."

As I previously mentioned, HDLs and LDLs are neither good nor bad. They are essential molecules that serve to transport cholesterol and fat throughout the body. Conventional medicine has spent too much time and money debating which is good and which is bad. Now, they are focused on the particle sizes of HDLs and LDLs. I feel this is more wasted time and money. Our health care dollars would be better used examining what is causing heart disease in the first place. High LDLs do not cause heart disease. Small LDL particle size does not cause heart disease. They are simply warning lights that something is wrong in the body.

SHOULD YOU TEST FOR HDL'S AND LDL'S?

The answer to that question is…maybe. An elevated LDL-cholesterol level is associated with an elevated risk of a heart disease. However, I believe the elevated LDL-cholesterol level is an innocent bystander doing what the body is asking it to do: bringing cholesterol to the tissues.

Infections lead to inflammation in the body. Perhaps the body is increasing its production of cholesterol and LDLs to help fight inflammation. The correct course in this case is to identify what is causing the inflammation and develop an appropriate treatment plan around that.

An elevated LDL-cholesterol level can also be an indicator of an infectious problem in the body. And, infections are known to be associated with heart disease. Furthermore, an elevated LDL-cholesterol level can indicate a metabolic problem in the body like diabetes. Both diabetes and infections are pro-inflammatory in the body and will increase inflammatory markers.

I do not believe that an elevated LDL-cholesterol blood

test warrants treatment with a cholesterol-lowering medication. Chapter 5 will show you that, at best, the use of statin medications to lower cholesterol and LDL-cholesterol levels has a 1-3.5% lowered risk for preventing a heart attack after taking the medication for approximately 3-5 years, which is the length of most studies. That means there is a 97-99% failure rate when using a statin medication to lower cholesterol and LDL-cholesterol levels in order to prevent heart disease. The efficacy of statin drugs is poor, especially when the drugs used are associated with serious adverse effects and are expensive. Furthermore, the safety of lowering LDL-cholesterol levels to target levels has never been determined.[19] And, finally, LDL target levels have never been shown to decrease mortality.[20] I predict PCSK9 medications will share a similar fate: They will not be shown to significantly decrease all-cause mortality or heart disease. In other words, the new PCSK9 medicines will lower LDL-cholesterol levels but not lower mortality rates significantly. In fact, I believe they will increase morbidity and mortality rates.

WHY DON'T THE MEDICINES THAT RAISE HDL-CHOLESTEROL AND LOWER LDL-CHOLESTEROL LOWER MORTALITY LEVELS?

That question is easy to answer: Because the whole model of heart disease is wrong. It is important to repeat that LDLs and HDLs are neither good nor bad. They are simply essential transport molecules for cholesterol and fat. We cannot live without either LDLs or HDLs.

When LDLs and cholesterol levels are elevated, an astute health care provider should be asking themselves, "Why are they elevated?" Instead, most conventional practitioners simply resort to using a drug therapy that poisons the pathway for the production of cholesterol and, eventually, LDL-cholesterol since it will parallel total cholesterol. Using a drug which lowers these levels is fine–if the elevated levels are causing the problems. However, elevated LDL-cholesterol and cholesterol do not cause any problems. They are simply bystanders doing what the body is calling for.

What raises cholesterol and LDL-cholesterol levels? Infections, metabolic disorders such as eating a poor diet, obesity, diabetes, hormone imbalances such as hypothyroidism, as well as toxicities and inflammation can all raise the levels. In this case, the astute practitioner will search for the underlying cause of the hypercholesterolemia and treat it. The worst case scenario in this situation is to use a drug that blocks cholesterol production as this does not address the underlying cause of the problem.

WHAT IS AN ELEVATED LDL AND CHOLESTEROL LEVEL?

That is the million dollar question. Conventional medicine

states that a cholesterol level over 200mg/dl and LDL-cholesterol greater than 100mg/dl are a problem. Newer recommendations are to further reduce the cholesterol and LDL levels even lower. I can summarize the new guidelines in one word: Ridiculous. They are based on studies showing very little benefit from statin medications and the guidelines ignore the cost and the toxicity of these medications. These artificial levels are nothing more than a clever marketing plan to gather more patients who need to be prescribed statin drugs.

I predict (discussed in Chapter 8) the new guidelines will not succeed in markedly lowering the rate of heart disease. Why should they? Statins have never been shown to markedly lower the rate of heart disease.

What is true is that half of all people suffering from a heart attack have low LDL-cholesterol levels—below 100mg/dl.[21] That means that half of the people who have heart attacks have high cholesterol levels. Other studies have shown no correlation with elevated lipid parameters—which include total cholesterol and LDL-cholesterol—and heart attacks.[22] However, many studies have shown an inverse correlation with cholesterol and LDL-cholesterol levels and heart disease—that means a lowered cholesterol/LDL level is associated with more heart disease.

I feel a lipid panel can be useful only when it is integrated with other blood work including hormone and nutrient levels as well as testing for inflammation, infection, blood viscosity (thickness), and heavy metals. As previously stated, cholesterol (which parallels LDL-cholesterol numbers) has anti-inflammatory properties. In times of inflammation, cholesterol levels will naturally rise to help the body protect the cells and put out the inflammatory fires. In this situation, an elevated cholesterol level neither represents a disease nor a need for a cholesterol-lowering medication.

FINAL THOUGHTS

If someone has elevated cholesterol due to a statin-deficiency syndrome, then I say treat them with a statin medication. However, in over 20 years of treating patients, I have yet to see a patient suffering from a statin-deficiency syndrome.

Elevated cholesterol and LDL levels are not the cause of cardiac illness; they may be the indicators of something else wrong such as a hormonal imbalance, infection, heavy metal toxicity or nutrient imbalances. Elevated cholesterol and LDLs are indications of inflammation. When they are found to be elevated, a thorough search should be undertaken to ascertain what is driving the inflammatory state. Only when the underlying cause of elevated cholesterol and LDL-cholesterol levels is determined can a treatment plan be implemented.

The following chapters of this book will address the underlying causes of elevated cholesterol and LDL levels.

[1] Accessed 11.28.14 from: http://www.heart.org/HEARTORG/Conditions/Cholesterol/AboutCholesterol/About-Cholesterol_UCM_001220_Article.jsp
[2] Advanced Nutrition and Human Metabolism, 6th Edition. Gropper and Smith. 2013. P. 172-173
[3] Infect. Immun. 57.p. 2237. 1989
[4] Infect. Immun. 61. P. 5140. 1993
[5] Cell Host & Microbe **4** (6): 555–66.
[6] J.Clin. Invest. Vol. 97. n.6. p. 1366-72. March, 1996.
[7] J. Clin. Invest. 62:1313=24. 1978
[8] Circ. Shock. 40:14-23. 1993
[9] Infect. Immun. 63:2401-6. 1995
[10] J. Acquir Immune Defic. Syndr. Hum. Retroviol. 17. P.51. 1998
[11] Circulation. 86(3):1046-60. 1992
[12] Lancet. 1:868-870. 1989
[13] J. of American Geriatrics Society. 53:219-26. 2005
[14] Innate Immunity December 2000 vol. 6 no. 6 421-430
[15] Lancet. 2007; **370**: 1829–1839
[16] JAMA. 2009; **302**: 1993–2000
[17] Lancet. Volume 380, No. 9841, p572–580, 11 August 2012
[18] *BMJ* 2014;349:g4379 doi: 10.1136/bmj.g4379
[19] Circ Cardiovasc Qual Outcomes. 2012;5:2-5.)
[20] Ann Intern Med. 2010;152:69 –
[21] Am. Heart J. Vol. 157 (1). p. 111-17. 2009
[22] JAGS 52:1639–1647, 2004

Chapter 4

Cholesterol: What Is It Good For?

CHAPTER 4: INTRODUCTION

My experience has clearly shown that almost every patient who sees a cardiologist for any heart disease-related complaint is put on a cholesterol-lowering medication at the first visit, regardless of what his/her cholesterol levels are. It is almost as if conventional physicians are compelled to use their prescription pad at each visit. In the history of medicine, cholesterol-lowering medications are the most profitable drugs for Big Pharma. It is not only cardiologists that are prescribing these medications—family doctors, internists, and nearly all other primary care providers are also very busy writing prescriptions for statin medications. In 2010, more than 255 million prescriptions for statins and other lipid lowering drugs were filled in the U.S.[1] Why are so many prescriptions written? The number one reason is that Big Pharma currently spends more money on promotion than it does on research and development. In fact, a recent research study estimated that Big Pharma spends over 19-fold more money on promotion versus discovering new molecules.[2] This number should not be a shock to anyone who watches television and sees the number of Big Pharma ads that are shown.

CHOLESTEROL: A DANGEROUS SUBSTANCE?

With the number of cholesterol-lowering medications being prescribed, no one could fault you for thinking that cholesterol is a dangerous substance. It must be so dangerous that new cardiovascular guidelines recommend that nearly every adult over the age of 65, both men and women, should be treated with cholesterol-lowering medications.[3] In fact, the recent guidelines recommend that 100% of men and 97% of everyone between the ages of 66 to 75 should be prescribed a statin drug. And, unbelievably, there are new guidelines to treat children as young as eight years old with statin drugs even though there are no randomized trials of children proving that statin drugs are safe.[4] Knowing how important cholesterol is to the growing brain—the highest concentration of cholesterol in the body is found in the brain—should make it easy to proclaim that children should never be prescribed cholesterol-lowering medications.

Most health care providers believe that cholesterol is responsible for clogging up the coronary arteries causing the epidemic of heart disease that has been occurring for over 70 years. I call this the "cholesterol = heart disease" hypothesis. If you believe this hypothesis, then you must assume that cholesterol is a dangerous substance which must be strictly controlled.

However, I have news for you: Cholesterol is an extremely important substance that we cannot live without. In other words, life itself is not possible without adequate amounts of cholesterol in the body.

If cholesterol is so important for each and every cell in body, it must have positive effects. However, in order to inflate the number of cholesterol-lowering medications being prescribed, The Powers-That-Be do not want you to be aware of what the beneficial effects of cholesterol are. In this chapter, I will educate you on why you need to ensure that you have adequate cholesterol production in the body.

This chapter can be summarized in the following bullet points:

- Cholesterol is needed by every single cell in the body both for function and reproduction.

- There is an inverse relationship between high cholesterol levels and the elderly; the higher the cholesterol level, the longer the life span.
- Half the people who die from a heart attack have high cholesterol levels; that means half who die have low cholesterol levels.
- Low cholesterol levels are associated with an increased risk for cancer.

CHOLESTEROL AND THE ELDERLY

It is important to keep in mind that over 90% of cardiovascular events occur in the elderly—people over the age of 65. And, many elderly currently take a statin medication. Over 48% of U.S. adults aged 75 and over currently take a statin medication.[5] However, in the elderly, the studies are clear; high cholesterol is *not* a risk factor for cardiovascular disease. When you factor in that there is no relationship in women between high cholesterol levels and the development of cardiovascular disease, only a small percentage of heart attacks can be related to high cholesterol levels. Even that argument is spurious as an association does not necessarily imply causation. Remember, in order for a hypothesis to be true, it has to withstand all counterarguments. The facts above clearly prove that the cholesterol = heart disease hypothesis is simply a false hypothesis.

ELEVEN IMPORTANT FUNCTIONS OF CHOLESTEROL

The key question for this chapter is, "What is cholesterol good for?" I will provide you with eleven crucial functions of cholesterol.

1. In the elderly, longevity increases with increased cholesterol Levels

Every person over the age of 65 should understand this: the higher your cholesterol level is the longer you will live. My friend and colleague, Uffe Ravnskov, M.D. has been lecturing and writing about this phenomenon for years. Dr. Ravnskov's book, **_The Cholesterol Myths_**, cannot be recommended highly enough.

There are dozens of studies which have reported that higher cholesterol levels are not associated with an increased mortality or an increase in cardiovascular disease.[6] (Thank you to Uffe Ravnskov, M.D., for putting much of this information together). Furthermore, many studies show an inverse correlation with cholesterol levels and longevity; the higher the total cholesterol level, the longer the longevity.

2. Cholesterol Has Anti-Inflammatory Properties

Most health care practitioners fail to understand that cholesterol has potent anti-inflammatory properties. Cholesterol (via 25-hydroxycholesterol—a metabolite derived from cholesterol) has been shown to inhibit potent inflammatory molecules such as pro-interleukin-1β.[7] Other researchers reported that mice who lack the ability to produce 25-hydroxycholesterol produce increased amounts of pro-inflammatory cytokines.[8]

3. Cholesterol is a precursor molecule for the sex hormones

All the adrenal and sex hormones including DHEA, pregnenolone, progesterone, testosterone, and estrogen are produced downstream from cholesterol. My experience has clearly shown that patients with low cholesterol levels have low sex and adrenal hormone levels and many of them suffer from hypoadrenal and hypogonadal symptoms. It should be no surprise to know that research has shown that statin drugs significantly lower sex hormone levels.[9]

4. Cholesterol is necessary for proper cell functioning

Every cell needs adequate amounts of cholesterol for its replication. Without an adequate amount of cholesterol, the cell will die. This simple fact should call into question the wisdom of chemically lowering cholesterol levels with statin medications.

5. Cholesterol is needed for maintaining cell structure

Cholesterol is an integral substance in each one of the trillions of cell membranes in the human body. It is needed to maintain the strength of the cell membranes. The cell membrane is sometimes referred to as the "brain" of the cell since it decides what comes in and out of the cell. A damaged cell membrane will allow toxic elements to enter the cell.

6. Cholesterol is needed to make the myelin sheath that surrounds all the nerves of the body

Without adequate cholesterol levels, nerve tissue will suffer. This should be no surprise once you understand how important cholesterol is to myelin production Myelin disorders are associated with neurological conditions such as multiple sclerosis.

7. Brain synapses—the connections between nerve cells—need a large amount of cholesterol

The reason statin drugs are associated with brain dysfunction is due, in part, to depleting the brain of cholesterol. Again, it should be no surprise that low cholesterol levels are associated with depression, suicide, and cognitive impairment.

Many studies have shown that a lowering of serum cholesterol concentration in middle-aged subjects leads to an increase in deaths due to suicide or violence.[10] Compared to normal and psychiatric control subjects, cholesterol concentrations in suicide attempters were found to be significantly lower.[11]

8. **The brain depends on cholesterol for optimal functioning**

The highest concentration of cholesterol in the body is located in the brain. Poor brain function is a common adverse effect of medications that lower cholesterol levels. Statin drugs have been known to cause sudden memory loss and cognitive impairment.

9. **Bile is produced from cholesterol and is needed to digest and process fats**

Bile is needed to digest and break down fats as well as to absorb fat-soluble vitamins. Cholesterol is the precursor molecule for bile production. All of the cholesterol-lowering medications are associated with gastrointestinal disorders including the older (fibrate) and the newer (statin) medications.

10. Cholesterol is necessary to produce vitamin D

Inadequate cholesterol production will ensure suboptimal vitamin D levels. We are suffering from an epidemic of vitamin D deficiency that is due, in part, to an overuse of statin medications.

Vitamin D deficiency is associated with the development of cardiovascular disease.[12] The Framingham study found subjects free of cardiovascular disease at baseline had a 50-80% increased risk of developing cardiovascular disease if they had low vitamin D levels.[13] The National Health and Nutrition Examination Survey III (NHANES) of 13,331 adults found an inverse correlation with vitamin D and cardiovascular mortality. In other words, the lower the vitamin D levels, the higher the mortality from cardiovascular disease. In fact, they found a 26% (RR) increased mortality when those in the lowest quartile (<17.8ng/ml) of vitamin D were compared to those in the highest (>32.1ng/ml).

11. Babies Need Adequate Amounts of Cholesterol For Proper Neurological Development

Breast milk is rich in cholesterol for a reason; the growing child needs cholesterol for optimal neurological and immune system development. Nursing mothers should ensure that they have an adequate intake of cholesterol and fats in their diets. Needless to say, nursing and pregnant mothers should not take statin medications.

Final Thoughts

Cholesterol is not a dangerous substance. It is an essential element needed by every cell in the body. The elderly who have higher total cholesterol levels have a better statistical chance of living longer when compared to an elderly person with low cholesterol levels. That simple fact is enough to invalidate the cholesterol = heart disease hypothesis.

When you understand the wide-ranging effects that cholesterol has in the body, who would want to take a medication that poisons the cholesterol biosynthetic pathway?

We are suffering from an epidemic of hormonal imbalances, vitamin D deficiency, digestive problems, and memory issues. Could there be an underlying cause to these problems? It could be from the over-use of statin medications.

If someone has a statin-deficiency syndrome, I say a statin may be indicated for him/her. Otherwise, it is best to avoid taking a statin medication.

[1] Stone, Kathlyn. Accessed 2.1.15 from: http://pharma.about.com/od/Sales_and_Marketing/a/The-Most-Prescribed-Medications-By-Drug-Class.htm
[2] British Med. J. 2012;344:e4348 doi: 10.1136/bmj.e4348
[3] Eligibility for Statin Therapy According to New Cholesterol Guidelines and Prevalent Use of Medication to Lower Lipid Levels in an Older US Cohort: The Atherosclerosis Risk in Communities Study Cohort. JAMA Internal Medicine. Published online November 17, 2014.
[4] Circulation. 2007; 116: 594-595
[5] NCHS Data Brief. N. 177, December, 2014. Accessed 2.11.15 from: http://www.cdc.gov/nchs/data/databriefs/db177.htm
[6] Kozarevic D et al. Serum cholesterol and mortality: the Yugoslavia Cardiovascular Disease Study. Am J Epidemiol. 1981 Jul;114(1):21-8.

Rudman D, Mattson DE, Nagraj HS, Caindec N, Rudman IW, Jackson DL. Antecedents of death in the men of a Veterans Administration nursing home. J Am Geriatr Soc. 1987 Jun;35(6):496-502. Forette B, Tortrat D, Wolmark Y. Cholesterol as risk factor for mortality in elderly women. Lancet. 1989 Apr 22;1(8643):868-70.

Staessen J, Amery A, Birkenhager W, Bulpitt C, Clement D, de Leeuw P, Deruyttere M, De Schaepdryver A, Dollery C, Fagard R, et al. Is a high serum cholesterol level associated with longer survival in elderly hypertensives? J Hypertens. 1990 Aug;8(8):755-61.

Harris T, Feldman JJ, Kleinman JC, Ettinger WH Jr, Makuc DM, Schatzkin AG. The low cholesterol-mortality association in a national cohort. J Clin Epidemiol. 1992 Jun;45(6):595-601.

Casiglia E et al. Predictors of mortality in very old subjects aged 80 years or over.

Eur J Epidemiol. 1993 Nov;9(6):577-86.

Krumholz HM, Seeman TE, Merrill SS, Mendes de Leon CF, Vaccarino V, Silverman DI, Tsukahara R, Ostfeld AM, Berkman LF. Lack of association between cholesterol and coronary heart disease mortality and morbidity and all-cause mortality in persons older than 70 years. JAMA. 1994 Nov 2;272(17):1335-40.

Weverling-Rijnsburger AW, Jonkers IJ, van Exel E, Gussekloo J, Westendorp RG. High-density vs low-density lipoprotein cholesterol as the risk factor for coronary artery disease and stroke in old age. Arch Intern Med. 2003;163(13):1549-54.

Jonsson A, Sigvaldason H, Sigfusson N. Total cholesterol and mortality after age 80 years. Lancet. 1997 Dec 13;350(9093):1778-9

Räihä I, Marniemi J, Puukka P, Toikka T, Ehnholm C, Sourander L. Effect of serum lipids, lipoproteins, and apolipoproteins on vascular and nonvascular mortality in the elderly. Arterioscler Thromb Vasc Biol. 1997 Jul;17(7):1224-32.

Behar S et al. Low total cholesterol is associated with high total mortality in patients with coronary heart disease. The Bezafibrate Infarction Prevention (BIP) Study Group. Eur Heart J. 1997 Jan;18(1):52-9.

Fried LP, Kronmal RA, Newman AB, Bild DE, Mittelmark MB, Polak JF, Robbins JA, Gardin JM. Risk factors for 5-year mortality in older adults: the Cardiovascular Health Study. JAMA. 1998 Feb 25;279(8):585-92.

Chyou PH, Eaker ED. Serum cholesterol concentrations and all-cause mortality in older people. Age Ageing. 2000 Jan;29(1):69-74.

Schatz IJ, Masaki K, Yano K, Chen R, Rodriguez BL, Curb JD. Cholesterol and all-cause mortality in elderly people from the Honolulu Heart Program: a cohort study. Lancet. 2001 Aug 4;358(9279):351-5.

Weverling-Rijnsburger AW, Jonkers IJ, van Exel E, Gussekloo J, Westendorp RG. High-density vs low-density lipoprotein cholesterol as the risk factor for coronary artery disease and stroke in old age. Arch Intern Med. 2003;163(13):1549-54.

Onder G, Landi F, Volpato S, Fellin R, Carbonin P, Gambassi G, Bernabei R. Serum cholesterol levels and in-hospital mortality in the elderly. Am J Med. 2003;115(4):265-71.

Casiglia E, Mazza A, Tikhonoff V, Scarpa R, Schiavon L, Pessina AC. Total cholesterol and mortality in the elderly. J Intern Med. 2003 Oct;254(4):353-62.

Psaty BM, Anderson M, Kronmal RA, Tracy RP, Orchard T, Fried LP, Lumley T, Robbins J, Burke G, Newman AB, Furberg CD. The association between lipid levels and the risks of incident myocardial infarction, stroke, and total mortality: The Cardiovascular Health Study. J Am Geriatr Soc. 2004 Oct;52(10):1639-47.

Ulmer H, Kelleher C, Diem G, Concin H. Why Eve is not Adam: prospective follow-up in 149650 women and men of cholesterol and other risk factors related to cardiovascular and all-cause mortality.J Womens Health 2004 Jan-Feb;13(1):41-53.

Schupf N, Costa R, Luchsinger J, Tang MX, Lee JH, Mayeux R. Relationship between plasma lipids and all-cause mortality in nondemented elderly. J Am Geriatr Soc. 2005 Feb;53(2):219-26.

Akerblom JL, Costa R, Luchsinger JA, Manly JJ, Tang MX, Lee JH, Mayeux R, Schupf N. Relation of plasma lipids to all-cause mortality in Caucasian, African-American and Hispanic elders. Age Ageing. 2008;37:207-13.

Newson RS et al. Association between serum cholesterol and noncardiovascular mortality in older age. J Am Geriatr Soc. 2011;59:1779-85
[7] NEJM. Nov. 13, 2014. 371;20. 1933-5
[8] Science 8 August 2014:
Vol. 345 no. 6197 pp. 679-684
[9] Urology. 76(5), 2010. p. 1048-105
[10] The Lancet. Vol. 339:8795. 3.21. 1992. 727-9
[11] Biol. Psychiatry. Vol. 41:2. 1.15.1997. 196-200
[12] J Am Coll Cardiol 2008;52:1949–56
[13] Circulation 2008;117:503–11

Chapter 5

The Cholesterol = Heart Disease Hypothesis

CHAPTER 5: INTRODUCTION

Death from cardiovascular disease is the number one killer in the U.S. It is estimated that 810,000 Americans die each year from heart diseases and stroke.[1]

As I mentioned before, when I was in medical school, I was taught that cholesterol was a dangerous substance. Furthermore, I was told that cholesterol was responsible for the heart disease and stroke epidemic and that I should consider using medications to lower cholesterol levels in all patients suffering from cardiovascular disease. Moreover, I was taught that the lower the cholesterol, the better outcomes my patients would have. Recently, this message was reiterated and expanded by the 2013 cholesterol guidelines which recommend putting nearly everyone on cholesterol-lowering medications in order to help prevent/treat heart disease.

At my graduation from Wayne State University School of Medicine, I remember when the dean told my class, "We have just taught you the most up-to-date medical information that is available. Unfortunately, about 50% of what you have learned is wrong. It is up to you to figure out which of the 50% is incorrect."

After 20 years of practicing medicine and continually studying biochemistry, I think my dean needed to adjust his numbers. I think 75% of what I was taught in medical school was incorrect. And, well over 99% of the nutrition I was taught was incorrect. Finally, what I was taught about cholesterol was nearly 100% incorrect. Remember, the medical school curriculum is tightly controlled by The Powers-That-Be. They have deemed nutrition unworthy of being taught in medical school.

THE CHOLESTEROL = HEART DISEASE HYPOTHESIS

When I use the term cholesterol = heart disease, I am referring to the currently accepted dogma that elevated cholesterol is responsible for causing the heart disease epidemic we are facing. However, many (if not most) cardiologists feel that any cholesterol level can cause heart disease. The cholesterol = heart disease hypothesis would also state that cholesterol levels have to be reduced to their lowest amounts possible. Of course, this can only occur with the use of cholesterol-lowering drugs such as statin medications. We have spent an untold amount of health care dollars on this flawed hypothesis. We have wasted more money than is imaginable treating this failed paradigm.

Heart disease is our number one killer and it has been number one for well over 70 years. The cholesterol = heart disease hypothesis is the prevailing view of conventional medicine and it has been for well over 50 years. Conventional medicine is convinced that occlusions of the coronary arteries are caused by cholesterol. Yes, cholesterol is found in coronary plaques, but blaming cholesterol for the plaque is similar to blaming firemen for causing house fires since firemen are present at nearly all house fires.

Cholesterol is not the underlying cause of coronary occlusions and heart disease. How can I make a statement like that?

If elevated cholesterol levels were responsible for causing the heart disease epidemic then all individuals who have suffered a heart attack should have elevated cholesterol levels. In fact, 50% of patients who suffer a heart attack have normal cholesterol levels. A British study found that among British men aged 40-59, the distribution of blood cholesterol concentrations in those who went on to develop coronary heart disease overlapped considerably with the distribution of those who did not.[2]

Researchers studied 1,200 patients with angina who underwent cardiac catheterization.[3] They found no correlation between cholesterol levels and the degree of stenosis. Another study found 75% of those hospitalized for a heart attack had low cholesterol levels.[4]

Furthermore, if elevated cholesterol levels were responsible for causing heart attacks then it should be a risk factor for people of all ages and for both sexes. However, there are numerous studies showing an inverse correlation with elevated cholesterol levels and coronary heart disease mortality and morbidity as well as all-cause mortality in people older than 70 years.[5] For women, there is no correlation with elevated cholesterol levels and mortality from heart disease.[6] In fact, women have higher cholesterol levels than men and have much less heart disease. More about women and heart disease can be found in Chapter 10.

WHERE DID IT ALL START

Remember, the cholesterol = heart disease hypothesis states that too much cholesterol in our diets causes a buildup of cholesterol and plaque in our arteries. This leads to atherosclerosis or hardening of the arteries. The end result of this process is an acute obstruction of coronary blood flow resulting in a heart attack, stroke or death.

If all were that simple...

To understand how it all started, let's go back in time to the beginning. Nikolai Anichkov was a Russian researcher who was interested in what was causing atherosclerosis. He performed an experiment on rabbits where he fed cholesterol to rabbits and the rabbits developed atherosclerotic plaques and had high cholesterol levels. The plaques in the rabbits were similar in appearance to the way human arteries appeared in those suffering from cardiovascular disease. At the end of his study, Dr. Anichkov theorized that high cholesterol was responsible for the atherosclerosis.[7]

The cholesterol = heart disease hypothesis picked up steam in the 1950s when an American scientist, Dr. Ancel Keys, published a paper that found cardiovascular disease was directly related to dietary fat intake.[8] In this paper was a graph which showed a linear correlation between mortality from heart disease and dietary fat intake. The famous graph that accompanied his paper is shown in Figure 1. Also in 1955, President Dwight Eisenhower suffered his first heart attack at age 64. He was told to follow a low-fat, low-cholesterol dietary regimen which was closely followed by the press. However, President Eisenhower's dietary changes were for naught; he suffered several more heart attacks and died from heart disease in 1969 at the age of 78.

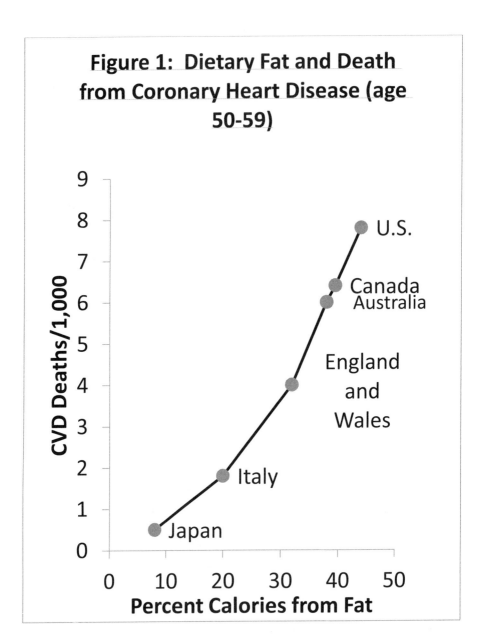

Adapted from Keys[9]

Looking at Figure 1, it is clear that there is a linear correlation between an increased intake of calories from fat and an increased cardiovascular disease death rate. Dr. Keys was very forceful in his lectures and he felt that his research proved beyond a doubt that dietary fat was responsible for the epidemic of cardiovascular disease that we were facing.

However, when Dr. Keys published his data—including his famous graph as shown in Figure 1 he had much more data available than what he presented. In fact, instead of the six countries illustrated in Figure 1, he actually had similar data from 22 countries available. In fact, Dr. Keys omitted the data from France where citizens are known to eat a high amount of dietary fat and yet have a low rate of cardiovascular disease.

The data from the 22 countries that were available to Dr. Keys are shown in Figure 2. As can be seen in Figure 2, there is actually no linear correlation between the amount of fat intake and the cardiovascular death rate.

So, why did Dr. Keys report the data as shown in Figure 1 and omit the rest of the data (shown in Figure 2) which was available to him? My best guess is that Dr. Keys cherry-picked the data that would support his hypothesis. Purposely omitting the other data points should be considered scientific fraud. It is amazing to me that so few have commented on Dr. Keys' fraud.

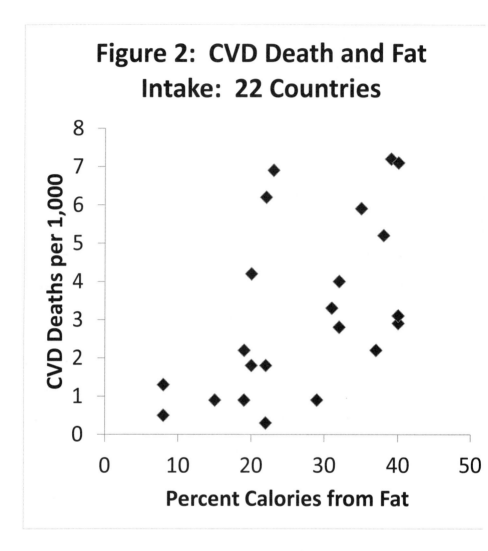

Figure 2: Adapted from Ravnoskov, Yerushalmy and Hilleboe[10]

A FLAWED HYPOTHESIS PICKS UP STEAM

Looking at all the data in Figure 2 clearly indicates that Dr. Keys' misrepresented the data available to him. By selectively using the data that would support his hypothesis, Dr. Keys concluded that elevated intake of dietary fat was directly related to the development of heart disease. Keys' conclusions were promoted by the American Heart Association, the U.S. Government, as well as nearly every other mainstream medical organization. Even 60 years later, most mainstream groups still agree with this failed hypothesis.

Dr. Keys lectured around the country about his findings. He promoted the idea that we needed to lower our intake of fatty foods in order to lower our rate of heart disease. The American Medical Association, the American Heart Association, nutritionists, the U.S. Government, and the rest of The Powers-That-Be bought into Dr. Keys' idea and recommended that all Americans switch to a low-fat diet. In fact, in 1957 margarine (made from vegetable oil) surpassed butter as the spread of choice.

THE PROMOTION OF LOW-FAT FOOD

In 1961, the American Heart Association raised 35 million dollars and officially adopted American Heart Association board member Ancel Keys' low-fat dietary recommendations.

In 1980, the U.S. Department of Agriculture released the first *Dietary Guidelines for Americans* which stated, on the cover, that we needed to "Avoid too much fat, saturated fat, and cholesterol".

In the mid to late 1980s, due to the Government's recommendations and the prevailing medical opinion from The Powers-That-Be, food manufacturers developed a plethora of low-fat foods that had low calorie counts. There were many choices of low-fat dairy products, vegetable oils, and other items that were promoted as heart-healthy. In fact, the American Heart Association still promotes this type of diet. Even today, on their website, they sell the *American Heart Association Low Fat, Low Cholesterol Cookbook*.[11]

Looking further into the American Heart Association website (www.heart.org), they state that we should "control hunger with filling foods that are low in calories." They recommend eating fat-free foods. They state, "High-fiber foods, such as fruits and vegetables, can provide a feeling of fullness and also digest slowly." My thoughts on their recommendations: This is nonsense. Foods that provide a sense of satiety are fat- and protein-containing foods. Carbohydrates do not provide a sense of satiety. More about diet and heart disease can be found in Chapter 14.

If the cholesterol = heart disease hypothesis was correct, as we lowered our intake of dietary fat and cholesterol, we should have seen heart disease incidence and mortality decline. That did not happen. Death from cardiovascular illness increased from 1900-1970, then started to decline which continued through 2010—see Figure 3.[12]

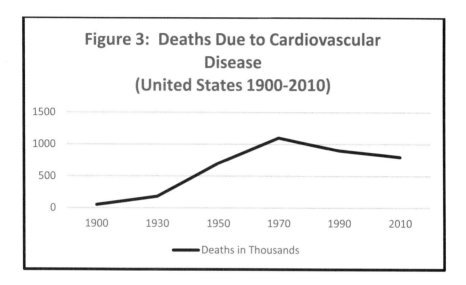

If physicians had studied earlier data, they would have rejected the hypothesis that cardiovascular disease was caused by eating too much dietary fat. For example, in England, from 1930-1955, the mortality from heart attacks increased six-fold while the intake of animal fat was unchanged.[13] In the U.S., dietary fat was relatively unchanged from the early 1900s until the mid to late 1980s when the consumption of low-fat foods dramatically increased—note from Figure 3, this change in fat consumption occurred after the decline of heart disease began. In fact, in nearly every country studied during these time periods, deaths from cardiovascular disease increased dramatically during the early part of the twentieth century independent of dietary fat changes.

THE NATIONAL CHOLESTEROL EDUCATION PROGRAM (1987)

In 1986-1987, to combat the nation's number one killer, the National Heart, Lung, and Blood Institute (NHLBI)—part of the National Institute of Health—announced a new program titled The National Cholesterol Education Program (NCEP). The National Cholesterol Education Program's goal was "To reduce the prevalence of elevated blood cholesterol in the United States and thereby contribute to reducing coronary heart disease morbidity and mortality."[14]

In the original report of the NCEP, it was stated, "For many, many years, the evidence identifying elevated blood cholesterol as a major risk factor for coronary heart disease has been well established. More recently, there has been a growing consensus that the reduction of elevated blood cholesterol can lead to a reduction in heart attacks and heart attack death. There are two factors that will be prominent in the development and implementation of this program. One is that it will be driven by science and the best collective judgment regarding the implications of scientific findings."

In effect, overnight, millions of Americans were suddenly told that they had a severe medical problem that required treatment. Patients were informed that the cause for heart disease had been determined and a treatment was available. The U.S. Government had thrown its enormous resources around the idea that all Americans needed to lower their cholesterol levels in order to prevent heart disease.

A 1987 article by T.J. Moore described it best. "One would expect a government program of such importance to have survived rigorous examination and review before it moved into high gear. One would suppose that such a far-reaching {medical} intervention into the lives of millions of people had been approved by the White House and scrutinized by Congress. In fact, the heart institute launched this project on its own authority, consulting panels of hand-picked specialists. One would suppose that before millions of people were put on such a medically supervised {program} it would have been tested to demonstrate that it was safe and effective. No such tests were conducted. In fact, laboratory performance was so poor that millions with average or low blood-cholesterol levels would inevitably be misled into believing that their levels were dangerously high."[15]

Keep in mind that before the proclamation that all high cholesterol levels were a risk factor for heart disease, heart disease mortality had been falling in the U.S. for the previous 10-

15 years. In fact, since 1970, the death rate from heart disease has fallen over 2.5x[16] (see Figure 4).

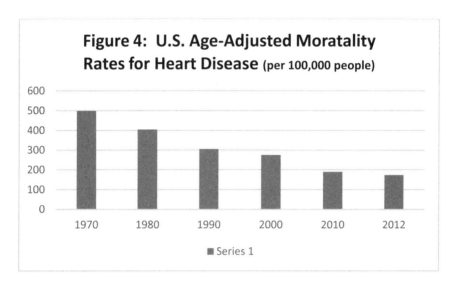

This decline started well before the discovery and use of cholesterol-lowering medications. Instead of beginning the NCEPs cholesterol-lowering campaign in 1987, researchers should have been asking why heart disease rates had been falling for almost 20 years previously. I am not sure if there is a single answer for why this decline occurred, but it is not due to falling cholesterol levels or the use of cholesterol-lowering medications.

Many researchers would have you believe that the use of statins is responsible for the declining rate of deaths from heart disease. They are wrong. Statins began to be widely used in the 1990s and beyond. Looking at Figure 4, it is clear that the age-adjusted mortality decline in deaths from heart disease cannot be attributed to statin use.

Final Thoughts

There is no consensus on what was responsible for the rapid rise of heart disease from 1930-1970. However, to blame too much cholesterol and fat in our diet is ludicrous. The studies, in total, have never shown that eating too many foods that contain cholesterol or dietary fat is responsible for the rapid increase in heart disease.

Similarly, there is no consensus on what caused the recent slight decline in deaths from heart disease – from 1970 to the present time. It is clear, however, that cholesterol-lowering medications are not responsible for the decline shown in Figure 3. Cholesterol-lowering medications were introduced in the 1980s and statins began to be used in large amounts in the mid-1990s—well after the decline in deaths which started in 1970. It is time conventional medicine stopped proclaiming that statins are responsible for this decline.

So what caused the decline? I am not sure, but the best bet may be the decline in cigarette smoking. Cigarette smoking is known to increase oxidative stress and inflammation. The decline in cigarette smoking parallels the decline in heart disease deaths shown in Figure 3.

[1] Accessed 12.1.14 from:
http://my.americanheart.org/professional/General/Trends-in-CVD-and-Stroke-Mortality_UCM_441066_Article.jsp
[2] BMJ. 3,7.1998. 316:723
[3] Atherosclerosis. 149(2000). p. 191-90
[4] American Heart Journal
Volume 157, Issue 1, January 2009, Pages 111–117.e2

[5] JAMA. Vol. 272"11.2.1994
[6] Circulation. Sep;86(3):1046-80. 1992
[7] Texas Heart Inst. J. 2006;33(4):417-23
[8] Journal of Mount Sinai Hospital. 20, 118-139. 1953
[9] Keys, A. Mt. Sinai Hospital. 20:118-139. 1953
[10] Ravnskov, Uffe. The Cholesterol Myths. 2000. Yerushalmyy and Hilleboe. New York State Journal of Medicine. 2343-2354. 1957
[11] Accessed 11.30.14 from:
http://www.heart.org/HEARTORG/GettingHealthy/NutritionCenter/Recipes/American-Heart-Association-Low-Fat-Low-Cholesterol-Cookbook-4th-Ed-Recipes_UCM_450562_Article.jsp
[12] As et al. Published online in Circulation Dec 18, 2013. Accessed 12.1.14 from: http://www.heart.org/idc/groups/heart-public/@wcm/@sop/@smd/documents/downloadable/ucm_449847.pdf
[13] The Lancet. 2. 155-162. 1957
[14] Public Health Reports. 1986. Jan-Feb 101(1). p. 2-3. Accessed 1.9.15 from: http://www.ncbi.nlm.nih.gov/pmc/articles/PMC1477656/
[15] The-Atlantic. Vol. 264. (25). Sept. 1989
[16] Accessed From the CDC (http://www.cdc.gov/nchs/data/databriefs/db168.htm) and American Heart Association (http://blog.heart.org/progress-against-heart-disease-stroke-reflected-in-latest-statistics/).

Chapter 6

The Biosynthetic Pathway for Cholesterol

CHAPTER 6: INTRODUCTION

In medical school, I learned that cholesterol was a dangerous substance. I was taught that cholesterol clogged the arteries and was responsible for the growing epidemic of our number one killer—heart attacks. Furthermore, I was instructed that the lower the cholesterol number, the better it would be for my patients.

Now, 25 years later, I can state with authority that what I was taught was wrong. Cholesterol is not a bad substance. It is a vital and necessary substance. In fact, the human body and the body of every living being requires adequate amounts of cholesterol not only to survive, but to thrive.

This chapter will focus on the biochemical pathways of cholesterol. For the non-scientists, you may think this is over your head. I assure you it is not. In order to understand why statin drugs cause such problems in the body, it is important to understand the cholesterol biochemical pathways. Only by understanding these pathways can you begin to see the dangers of statin medications. It does not take an advanced degree in biochemistry to understand this; it just takes some common sense. I will show you how cholesterol is produced and why it is essential for every single cell in the human body. In addition, I will review how cholesterol came to be demonized by The Powers-That-Be and how it continues to be misrepresented as a bad substance in today's modern world.

Cholesterol, Statins, and Biochemistry

To get into medical school, pre-med students must take a biochemistry course. In medical school, we are again taught biochemistry. You would think that most doctors would have a sound, fundamental understanding of biochemistry.

Unfortunately, most physicians do not understand biochemistry. If they did, more would reject many of the most-commonly used medications, including statins, due to their mechanism of action. Most prescription drugs—over 95%–work by disrupting the body's biochemical pathways. How do drugs do this? Drugs disrupt the biochemical pathways by poisoning enzymes or blocking receptors in the body.

In my book, *Drugs That Don't Work and Natural Therapies That Do*, I wrote about how the most common drugs are failing us. As compared to the rest of the world, Americans spend the most on health care. In fact, nearly 20% of our gross national product is spent on health care. The next major Western country (France) spends half that amount. Every other Western country spends less than half of what we spend. You would think we would have better outcomes for this huge expense. Well, you would think wrong. On every single health indicator, we rank last or near last. That includes outcomes from neonatal mortality to life-span.

Guess who spends the most on prescription drugs? The answer is not hard to come by. Americans take more prescription drugs and spend more on their medications than any people on the planet. Yet, we do not have fewer heart attacks, strokes or live longer than our Western friends. In reality, we have more heart attacks, strokes, and live shorter lives compared to the entire Western world.

In fact, we are spending too much money on ineffective and expensive drugs that do not provide enough positive results and at the same time are prone to serious adverse effects. In *Drugs That Don't Work and Natural Therapies That Do*, my basic premise states that it is impossible to poison a crucial enzyme or block an important receptor for the long term and expect a good result. This includes the most commonly-prescribed drugs which include:

- Statins for high cholesterol - poison the enzyme HMG-CoA reductase
- Proton pump inhibitors for blocking stomach acid production - poison the enzyme hydrogen/potassium adenosine triphosphatase enzyme system
- Bisphosphonates for treating osteoporosis - poison the enzyme farnesyl diphosphate synthase

I find it hard to believe that humans were designed to have their receptors blocked and their enzymes poisoned in order to be healthy. That doesn't make biochemical sense nor does it make common sense. Rather, physicians should be searching for the underlying cause of illness and using items that support and enhance the body's biochemistry.

How do you support biochemistry? Biochemical pathways are easily supported by providing the body with the basic nutrients it needs. This includes vitamins and minerals which all act as cofactors in the biochemical milieu.

THE BIOSYNTHETIC PATHWAY OF CHOLESTEROL

To review, cholesterol is a waxy substance that is found in

every cell in the body. In fact, no cell can survive without adequate amounts of cholesterol. It is produced in all animals but is not found in plants. In humans, the vast majority of cholesterol is produced in the liver.

The biosynthetic pathway for cholesterol production is complex and contains checks and balances to ensure that each and every cell of the body has an adequate supply of cholesterol (Figure 1). Unfortunately, most health care providers are ignorant of this pathway. I can state, with assurance, that if a health care provider is not knowledgeable about the biochemical pathway of cholesterol production, he or she cannot possibly begin to understand the importance of cholesterol production. Furthermore, if the health care provider is not up-to-date on the cholesterol biosynthetic pathway, he/she should not be prescribing a medication that impacts this pathway.

When I lecture to health care providers, I always show the biochemical pathways so that I can point out items that either support or inhibit these pathways. The human body was designed perfectly. In order for the body to function optimally, the human body must have available the raw materials which are necessary for the biochemical pathways to produce life-sustaining items such as energy in the form of adenosine triphosphate (ATP), proteins, hormones, etc. Understanding the pathways makes it easy to predict problems when the biochemistry is disrupted.

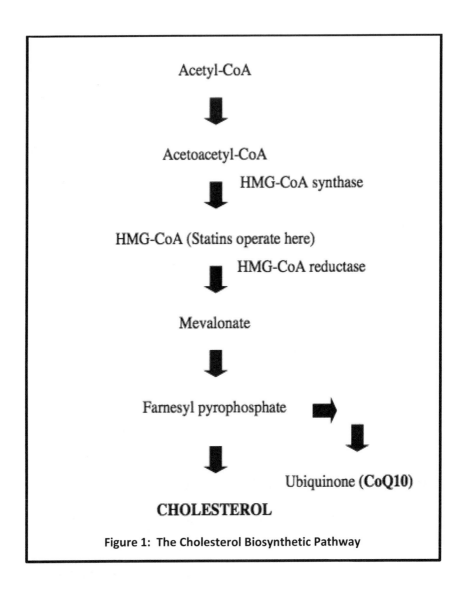

Figure 1: The Cholesterol Biosynthetic Pathway

The cholesterol biosynthetic pathway is necessary to produce many vital substances including hormones. More about these items are found in Chapter 11. For now, I will focus on how cholesterol is produced in the body.

Figure 1 shows some of the steps that are needed to produce cholesterol. The process starts from acetyl-CoA. Acetyl-CoA is used in many biochemical reactions. It is used for producing the energy molecule ATP in the Krebs cycle. Furthermore, Acetyl-CoA is the precursor molecule for fatty acid, glucose, and amino acid metabolism.

THE IMPORTANCE OF MEVALONATE

Each of the steps outlined in Figure 1 is important for normal cell function. Notice the molecule mevalonate in the middle of the pathway. Every cell depends on mevalonate for its life cycle. Without mevalonate, cells will die. Hannah (M.D.) and Yosef explain the importance of mevalonate in their book, *How Statin Drugs Really Lower Cholesterol.* They state, "Mevalonate is the essence of cell renewal. In all cells, mevalonate travels down the mevalonate pathway to make cholesterol and isoprenoids (five-carbon molecules). Both stimulate the cell to grow, replicate its DNA and divide into two cells. This is the "cell cycle". This is life. Without {downstream metabolites like isoprenyls—Farnesyl pyrophosphate} for DNA replication, there is no cell cycle. Without a cell cycle, cells age and die."[1] Isoprenoids are represented in Figure 1 as Farnesyl pyrophosphate.

Isoprenoids

Isoprenoids are made by both plants and animals. They are derived from five-carbon units and are a large class of organic compounds. Isoprenoids have a wide range of effects in plants including affecting growth, color, and odor of the plant. In plants, isoprenoids occur in the essential oils. In animals, isoprenoids are commonly found in the fatty areas and contribute to the yellow color of egg yolks.

In plants, isoprenoids are necessary to produce vital substances such as carotenoids–beta carotene and vitamin A. Furthermore, they are necessary to produce vitamins E and K1.

In humans, isoprenoids are precursor molecules needed for producing the vitamin-like substance CoQ10, dolichols, bile acids, and steroid hormones. (Figure 2). Humans cannot live without CoQ10 and the other isoprenoids produced in the cholesterol/mevalonate pathway. Unfortunately, cholesterol-lowering medications such as statin drugs poison the HMG-CoA reductase enzyme which ensures a lowered production of CoQ10, isoprenoids, dolichols, bile acids, and steroid hormones.

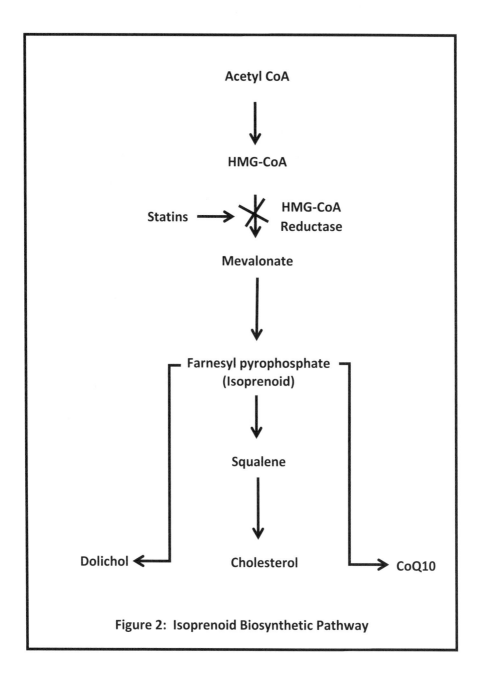

Figure 2: Isoprenoid Biosynthetic Pathway

DNA replication is also dependent on isoprenoid production.[2] This was first reported in 1980. The same researchers who reported this phenomenon also stated that mevalonate was required for DNA synthesis, cell growth, and replication.[3] Keep in mind, inhibiting cells from replication ensures their death. This is why statins cannot be used in pregnancy; isoprenoids are crucial for normal embryo development. Furthermore, isoprenoids are necessary for normal egg and sperm cell function. Once you understand the biochemical pathway of cholesterol production, you can see how statin medications are bound to cause adverse effects. More about the adverse effects of statins can be found in Chapter 9.

DOLICHOLS

As can be seen from Figure 2, dolichols are produced downstream from the isoprenoids. In fact, dolichols are produced in the same intermediate pathway that produces Coenzyme Q10.

Dolichols are important for linking together protein fragments into peptides. These peptides are important because they help the immune system function in cell identification and communication. Furthermore, these dolichol-induced peptides help anchor glycoproteins on the cell surface. Dolichols are also important molecules for DNA replication and repair. Without adequate dolichol production, DNA errors can accumulate. Too many DNA errors can lead to serious problems such as cancer. Knowing this, it should be no wonder that any drug that poisons the HMG-CoA reductase pathway has been shown to cause an increased risk of cancer. More about statins and the risk of cancer can be found in Chapter 9. In fact, there are many studies which have concluded that statin drug use is associated with an increased risk in cancer. [4] [5] [6] [7] [8] [9] Unfortunately, CoQ10 supplementation cannot reverse the inadequate production of dolichols.[10]

FINAL THOUGHTS

I find it fascinating to study the biochemical pathways. I am not sure why medical schools do not place more emphasis in the study of biochemistry. If they did, we would have a lot less illness and we would be spending much less on chronic disease care. It is important to note that medical schools do teach biochemistry to their students. However, they do not teach it in a clinically useful form. That needs to change. The only way doctors are going to learn about the importance of natural items such as vitamins and minerals is through the study of biochemistry.

The isoprenoids and the other intermediate substances in the mevalonate/cholesterol biosynthetic pathway make it clear that it is not wise to poison the mevalonate/cholesterol biosynthetic pathway. In fact, it does not take an advanced biochemistry degree to predict dire consequences from disrupting this important pathway. Since statin medications work by poisoning the HMG-CoA reductase enzyme in this pathway, it is no wonder that they are associated with a host of serious adverse side effects such as cancer, neuropathy, and myopathy.

[1] How Statin Drugs Really Lower Cholesterol and Kill You One Cell at a Time. 2012. p. 3.
[2] Proc. Natl. Acad. of Sci. USA. Vol. 77, N. 10. P. 5843-48. 1980
[3] IBID. How Statin Drugs Really Lower Cholesterol and Kill You One Cell at a Time. 2012. p. 9
[4] Arch. Int. Med. 153:1079-87. 1993
[5] J. Clin. Epidem. 56:280-5. 2003
[6] Int. J. Cancer. 114:643-7: 2005
[7] Br. J. Cancer. 2004:90:635-7
[8] J. Clin. Oncol. 2004:22:2388-94
[9] Cancer Epidemiol. Biomarkers Prev. 2007:16:4: 16-21
[10] Personal communication with Duanne Graveline, M.D., MPH.

Chapter 7

Statistics, Damn Statistics, and Statins

CHAPTER 7: INTRODUCTION

This chapter will review medical statistics and how they are used to over-inflate statin results.

For many years, future doctors have had to take a statistics class to get into medical school. I fulfilled that task during my undergraduate training at the University of Michigan. In medical school, we were again taught about statistics. You would think that most doctors are knowledgeable about statistics in order to be able to critically read research studies. However, if you think that most doctors understand statistics well enough to evaluate medical research articles, then you are incorrect. I would estimate that well over 95% of most physicians are incapable of critically reviewing any research article.

How can I make such a claim? I can state it because I used to be one of those doctors who could not properly evaluate scientific articles. As stated above, I took the required statistics courses in both my undergraduate and graduate medical training.

However, these courses were not taught in a way that I was able to understand the statistical methods that were—and are still—commonly used to write medical research articles. Furthermore, during that time in my career, I bought into what I was taught; I saw no reason to challenge my educators. I can guarantee you that nearly all practicing doctors and other health care providers are unprepared to understand how to critically evaluate a research study.

This chapter will show you how the vast majority of medical research is reported and how statistical methods are utilized to make this research look more positive than it truly is. The inaccurate reporting of research is supported and promoted by Big Pharma. The reason we use so many ineffective therapies, statin drugs included, is because of the statistical manipulation used in most medical research articles.

As I mentioned in Chapter 2, at my office, I have medical students, residents, other health professionals as well as practicing doctors shadow me for a period of time. I enjoy teaching other health professionals what I do in my practice of medicine. At the first visit to my office, every health professional is given a medical article. I ask them to read the article and report whether the therapy that the article is reporting on is successful or not.

Inevitably, everybody reports back to me what was in the abstract of the article. However, the abstract of nearly all research articles utilizes inaccurate statistical methods to report the data. The inaccurate statistical methods are utilized (in most cases) to provide a positive outcome about a therapy when the therapy is truly not very effective.

STATINS: PRIMARY VERSUS SECONDARY PREVENTION

Before we move on to the statistical analysis discussion, I must clarify some terms. I know this was done previously, but it is important to understand this concept. Statin studies inevitably report on cardiac outcomes. These outcomes can be referred to as primary and secondary prevention. Primary prevention refers to the prevention of the first cardiac event. Secondary prevention refers to a patient who has already suffered a cardiac event and is trying to prevent a second event.

A doctor who tells his/her patient to use a statin to prevent a first heart attack is using the statin for primary prevention. Big Pharma has a huge financial interest to promote statins for primary prevention as that would capture millions of healthy individuals who have not suffered a cardiac event. More about this later.

On the other hand, a health care provider who is prescribing a statin medication to a patient who has already suffered a heart attack or who already has heart disease is using the medication for secondary prevention. They are trying to prevent a secondary or recurrent event.

RELATIVE RISK VERSUS ABSOLUTE RISK

"Relative risk" (RR) is the term for a statistical analysis of data that is used to compare risk in two different populations over a time period. In other words, it is the ratio of the probability of developing a disease, or an event occurring in an exposed group compared to the probability of the event occurring in a non-exposed group. Big Pharma companies prefer to use such an analysis in their studies because the relative risk makes a treatment seem more effective than it really is. I would estimate that over 99% of most research articles reported in major medical journals are reported in relative risk terms. It has only been recently that a few medical papers report the more accurate term absolute risk (explained below) along with the relative risk.

- RR of 1 means there is no difference between the two groups.
- RR <1 means the event (or disease) is less likely to occur in the treatment group.
- RR >1 means the event is more likely to occur in the exposed group.

The relative risk can be calculated by using the following formula:

$$RR = \frac{\text{\% events in exposed or treatment group}}{\text{\% events in non-exposed or control group}}$$

What nearly all health professionals do not understand is that relative risk ratios were never meant to be used by a treating physician to determine if a particular therapy is useful for a patient.

ABSOLUTE RISK DIFFERENCE

The absolute risk (AR) difference is a better statistical representation of data that can be used by a health professional to decide if a specific therapy is useful for a patient. It is the absolute risk difference in event rate between a treatment group and a control group. Simply put, you can subtract the percentages affected in the treatment group from the control group to ascertain the AR difference. As reported in the New England Journal of Medicine, "Absolute differences in risk are more clinically important than relative reductions in risk in deciding whether to recommend a drug therapy."[1]

When I ask any medical student, resident, or any health professional to explain the difference between absolute and relative risk, they inevitably fail to do so. It is my premise that if a health professional cannot understand and calculate the absolute risk difference in a study then they cannot properly decide if that therapy is appropriate for a patient.

NUMBER NEEDED TO TREAT

I have one last statistical term to share with you. It is known as the number needed to treat (NNT). It is calculated by the following formula: 1/AR.

It is a helpful number for health care professionals to understand as it refers to the number of patients needed to treat with a drug (or a particular therapy) in order to achieve a desired result. Why is the NNT so important? If the NNT is very high, it suggests that the drug is ineffective. For example, a NNT of 100 refers to 100 people needing to be treated with a drug to prevent one from getting the illness. That means that 99 treated with the drug did not achieve the benefit of the drug. Another way to think about it is a NNT of 100 means that the drug failed 99% of people who took it and only one person out of one hundred (1%) was helped.

A better drug therapy would have a low NNT. A NNT of 1 means that for every patient treated with the drug, all are cured of the disease the drug was designed to treat. Effective NNT treatments are in the range of 1-4. A NNT over 20—means the drug is virtually worthless as 19 out of 20 took the drug without getting the desired result. That is a 95% failure rate (19/20).

There are only two drugs with a NNT of 1, meaning every patient treated with that drug for that condition has a positive result. The drugs are insulin for Type 1 diabetics and thyroid hormone for hypothyroidism.

STATINS FAIL OVER 99% WHO TAKE THEM

Nearly all statin studies have a NNT of at least 100 and many are in the 200-300 range. That means that 99% of those that take statins receive no benefit. This alone should cause The Powers-That-Be to stop recommending statins for so many.

LET'S PUT IT ALL TOGETHER: A HYPOTHETICAL RESEARCH STUDY

I will compose a fake drug research study where 100 subjects are in the treatment group (treated with Drug X) and 100 subjects are in the placebo group. Both are followed for three years. The end point is a heart attack. In this study, two people in the placebo group had a heart attack versus one in the treatment group—see Table 1 below. I will calculate the RR, AR, and the NNT.

Table 1: Hypothetical Drug Research Study 200 Subjects

	Heart Attacks (number)	Percent Suffering Heart Attack
Drug Treatment	1	1%
Placebo	2	2%

The relative risk reduction (RR) is 1%/2%=0.5. The headlines could shout, "Drug X Provides Fifty Percent Reduction in Heart Attacks."

However, the absolute risk reduction (AR) is 2%-1%=1%. More truthful headlines should state, "Drug X Provides a 1% Benefit in Preventing Heart Attacks."

The number needed to treat (NNT) is 1/0.01 or 100. Therefore, this study showed that 100 people would need to be treated for three years (the length of the study) to prevent one heart attack. A knowledgeable health care provider should tell his patient that this drug failed 99% who took it, since 99 out of 100 received no benefit.

Now, let's do the same three year study with 1,000 patients in both the treatment and the placebo group. Similarly to the previous 100 patient study, two people in the control group suffered a heart attack as compared to one in the treatment group. The results are shown in Table 2 below.

Table 2: Hypothetical Research Study 2000 Subjects

	Heart Attacks (number)	Percent Suffering Heart Attack
Drug Treatment	1	0.1%
Placebo	2	0.2%

The RR is the same as the previous hypothetical study (Table 1): 0.1%/0.2%=0.5. The media headlines could state the same: "Drug X Provides a Fifty Percent Reduction in Heart Attacks."

Here, the AR is different. 0.2%-0.1%=0.1%. More truthful headlines should read, "Drug X Provides a 0.1% Benefit in Preventing Heart Attacks." The NNT has also worsened:

1/0.1%=1,000. Therefore, a health care provider should educate their patient that 1,000 patients needed to be treated with Drug X in order to prevent one heart attack. Therefore, the drug is a 99.9% failure as 999 out of 1,000 patients did not gather any heart attack benefit.

You could see what would happen if I expanded the study to 10,000 subjects or more.

If Drug X had no side effects and was inexpensive, it might be worthwhile for someone to take it to prevent a heart attack even though it was only 1% effective. However, if the drug is associated with adverse effects and is expensive, then one should consider calling drug X what it is: A failure.

STATINS AND RELATIVE RISK

I would estimate that nearly 100% (perhaps I have missed one) of the published statin articles report their data in a relative risk format. Most statin studies have compared groups of patients who have taken a statin medication with a similar group that has not taken a statin drug.

Let's go back in time to 2005 when statin drugs were beginning to be used in millions of patients. One of the famous articles promoting the use of statins appeared in the American Journal of Medicine.[2] This article reported on the Anglo-Scandinavian Cardiac Outcomes Trial (ASCOT). ASCOT was the first trial of statin medications used to assess the benefits of cholesterol lowering in the primary prevention of coronary heart disease in patients with hypertension who were not deemed to have dyslipidemia (abnormal lipid testing) by conventional measures.

A total of 19,342 patients with hypertension and greater than three risk factors for heart disease (such as diabetes, obesity, smoking, etc.,), but without heart disease, were enrolled in ASCOT. Of these, 10,305 patients with a serum cholesterol level of <250mg/dl were randomized to either atorvastatin (Lipitor—10mg/day) or a placebo. As reported in the abstract of the article, "The trial was stopped early—3.3 years instead of the planned five years—due to the superiority of {Lipitor} 10mg over placebo in reducing the primary end point of nonfatal and fatal myocardial infarction by 36%." The 36% decline in heart attacks reported in the abstract was a relative risk number.

Remember, a relative risk number should not be used when deciding whether a therapy is appropriate for a particular patient. The absolute risk difference is needed for that decision—and the absolute risk difference was not reported in this study. In order to understand what the absolute risk difference of this study was one would have to manually calculate this number from the data in the article.

This is exactly what I ask all the students to do when they come to my office---calculate and explain the absolute risk reduction in a study. Before I show you how to calculate the absolute risk reduction, let me tell you what Big Pharma charter member (I made up the charter member designation) Pfizer did with the results of this study.

Pfizer spent more than $258 million advertising Lipitor—with most of this advertising budget used to promote ASCOT. Ads were seen in print—in magazines and newspapers as well as on television.[3] A copy of the most widely used print ad is seen below.

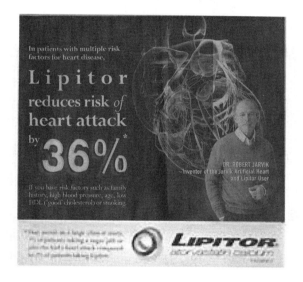

Pfizer used the likeness of Dr. Robert Jarvik as a spokesman for its Lipitor campaign. Dr. Jarvik was a pioneer in the development of the artificial heart pump.

This ad came under scrutiny from the United States House Energy and Commerce Committee for false advertising as one ad showed Dr. Jarvik rowing a boat when it wasn't actually him rowing the boat. The House committee forced Pfizer to stop using Dr. Jarvik in their ads. I was happy Pfizer was forced to remove the ads, but I thought the ads should have been removed for failing to report the true reduction in heart disease that was shown in that study: 1%.

WHEN IS A HEART ATTACK REDUCTION OF 36% REALLY 1%?

What do I mean by false advertising? You can see from this ad that it states, "In patients with multiple risk factors for heart disease, Lipitor reduces the risk of heart attack by 36% if you have risk factors such as family history, high blood pressure, age, low HDL, or smoking."

Heart disease is our number one killer. Anything that reduces the risk of heart disease by 36% would garner my attention and it should garner yours.

When I looked at the data from the study, I quickly realized that the 36% reduction was a relative risk calculation. Let me show you the data. There were two groups studied in ASCOT: A treatment group of 5,168 subjects treated with Lipitor and a control group of 5,137 treated with a placebo. Table 3 below summarizes the information about how the two groups fared during the study period.

Table 3: ASCOT Study

ASCOT Study	Number of fatal coronary heart disease and non-fatal myocardial infarction	% suffering fatal coronary heart disease and non-fatal myocardial infarction
Lipitor	100	2%
Placebo	154	3%

If you look closely at the Jarvik Lipitor ad on page 107, you will see an asterisk after the 36%. I always tell my students to follow the asterisks.

I have reprinted below the actual part of the ad which the asterisk points to. It states:

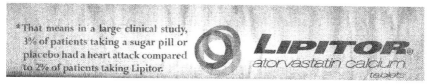

"*That means in a large clinical study, 3% of patients taking a sugar pill or placebo had a heart attack compared to 2% of patients taking Lipitor."

LIPITOR AND MANIPULATED STATISTICS

So, how did they get a 36% reduction from the above statement? Again, this is a perfect example of why it is so important to understand the difference between relative and absolute risk.

Let me show you how to do the calculations.

In the ASCOT study, there were 100 cardiac events in the treatment group out of 5,168 subjects. Therefore, 100/5168=0.019. In the placebo group, there were 154 events out of 5,137 subjects. Therefore, 154/5137=0.030.

To calculate the relative risk (RR), I can plug in the numbers below to show:

$$RR = \frac{0.019}{0.030} = 0.64 \text{ (rounded)}$$

Remember, a RR <1 confers benefit from the treatment. Therefore, the ASCOT study shows a 36% RR benefit: 1 - .64=.36=36%.

The 36% reduction is the statistical manipulation of the data that is known as the relative risk. As I stated previously, the RR is not meant to be used when making a decision whether a particular therapy is relevant to the patient sitting in front of them.

The most important number that the doctor can have available to him/her is the absolute risk difference. In fact, RR is completely meaningless without the AR numbers. The absolute risk difference is simply calculated by subtracting the percent difference in risk between the two groups. For example, in the ASCOT example above, the absolute risk difference is 3% minus 2%, which equals 1%. A more accurate headline in the Lipitor advertisement previously shown should have stated, "In patients with multiple risk factors for heart disease, Lipitor reduces the risk of heart attack by 1%, if you have risk factors such as family history, high blood pressure, age, low HDL, or smoking."

Therefore, a health care provider counseling his/her patient about whether taking a statin will significantly reduce their risk of developing a heart attack should state, according to the data from ASCOT, "You have a 1% lowered risk of developing a heart attack if you take Lipitor for 3.3 years." (The length of the study was 3.3 years.)

Furthermore, an accurate statement of the data from ASCOT is that Lipitor failed 99% who took it. How can I make that statement? If 1% of those studied had fewer heart attacks from taking Lipitor, what about the other 99% exposed to the drug? They did not receive the benefit. Furthermore, they had to pay for the drug and, by taking Lipitor, exposed themselves to adverse side effects.

I think that if patients were informed about the true numbers of this as well as other statin studies, far fewer patients would be willing to take a statin drug.

STATINS FAIL MOST WHO TAKE THEM

Right now, you are probably thinking to yourself that this cannot be true. Maybe the other studies show better results.

However, the opposite is true; all of the other statin studies fail to show significantly better results than ASCOT. The best of the statin studies show a 1-3.5% decline in death from heart attacks due to taking a statin medication for three to five years, which is the general length of most statin studies. Another way I can make my point is by saying that **statins fail 96.5-99% of those who take them**—they do not provide a reduced risk of death from a heart attack and they expose the patients to possible adverse effects from taking the drug.

The ASCOT study had a NNT of 100 (1/1% or 1/.01) which means that, according to ASCOT, 100 patients would need to take Lipitor for 3.3 years (the length of the study) to prevent one heart attack. This equates to a 99% failure rate of Lipitor as 99/100 took the drug without getting the benefit. They were exposed to possible adverse effects and had to pay for the Lipitor for three years. At the time of the study, Lipitor cost $140/month. To prevent one heart attack would cost nearly $600,000. I can think of better ways to spend this money.

JUPITER: ANOTHER FAILED STATIN STUDY

I could analyze any statin study and show you that the AR is around 1-2% and the NNT is at least 100. However, I would like to spend time on the JUPITER study as it was (and is) widely touted as a successful study for statin therapy, especially for healthy people. JUPITER is where The Powers-That-Be claim they show a primary prevention benefit for statin drugs.

Statins can be recommended for either primary or secondary prevention. As previously mentioned, primary prevention means a statin drug is recommended to prevent a first cardiac event. In other words, a patient has not had a heart attack or stroke. In contrast, secondary prevention with statin therapy refers to taking a statin medication to prevent a second cardiac event—in other words, the patient has already suffered a heart attack or stroke.

In conventional medicine, statins have had an indication for use in secondary prevention as many studies have shown that statins lower the risk of a heart attack by 1-3.5%. (Side note: I am not sure why a 1-3.5% decline in secondary heart attacks would warrant their use, but that is the way conventional medicine operates.)

The Big Pharma Cartel has been pining for a primary prevention benefit of statins as this would open up the market to millions of new patients—ones who have not had a cardiac event but would be encouraged to take statin medications. ASCOT was a secondary prevention study as many of these subjects had a previous cardiac event.

JUPITER was a study of 17,802 healthy men and women with LDL-cholesterol <130mg/dl and high-sensitivity C-reactive protein levels of >2.0mg/L. C-reactive protein is a blood test that, when elevated, is a sign of inflammation in the body. I am not sure why the authors stated that JUPITER was a study of 'healthy' men and women as an elevated C-reactive protein is a warning sign that these patients were suffering from an inflammatory condition.

The subjects were randomized into two groups: A placebo group and a treatment group who took 20mg of Crestor® daily. The endpoints of the trial were cardiovascular events including heart attack, stroke, hospitalization for unstable angina, arterial revascularization (coronary bypass surgery), or death from cardiovascular causes. The trial was set to run for five years, but was stopped at 1.9 years because the Crestor®-treated group had such "positive" results.

I remember when JUPITER was reported—in November, 2008. I opened up my morning papers—*The Wall Street Journal* (WSJ) and *The New York Times* (NYT)—and saw the bold headlines touting the positive results of JUPITER. The NYT article stated, "A large new study suggests that millions more people could benefit from taking the cholesterol-lowering drugs known as statins, even if they have low cholesterol, because the drugs can significantly lower their risk of heart attacks, strokes and death." The WSJ commented, "...Crestor® sharply lowered the risk of heart attacks among apparently healthy patients in a major study that challenges longstanding heart-disease prevention strategies." In *USA Today*, an article commenting on the results of JUPITER stated, "This is going to have huge repercussions. We know that we can reduce the risk of heart attack, stroke and angioplasty by nearly 50%." Other news outlets touted the results of JUPITER reporting a 50% reduction in heart attacks and a 20% decline in death in the treatment group.

When I read those articles, I remember wondering how this could be. I studied the statin research from the beginning and I knew that no study of healthy or sick people came close to these numbers. I wondered if I had been wrong; maybe this was the breakthrough study for statins that proved they worked in a majority of people.

When I went to my office that morning, I called the hospital librarian and requested the full JUPITER article. At lunch I read it and made my own calculations. After analyzing the data, I realized JUPITER was another failed statin study. Here's my analysis of JUPITER.

There were 8,901 subjects in the Crestor®-treated group and 8,901 in the placebo group.

Table 4 below shows the data from JUPITER. The number of people who suffered an event is shown with the percentages in parentheses.

Table 4: JUPITER RESULTS

	Crestor®	Placebo
Non-Fatal Heart Attacks	22 (0.25%)	62 (0.70%)
Fatal Heart Attack	9 (0.10%)	6 (0.07%)
Any Heart Attack	31 (0.35%)	68 (0.76%)
Death from any cause	198 (2.22%)	247 (2.78%)

How did the lay press come up with a 50% reduction in heart attacks? They used an RR number (0.35/0.76=50%). However, the more-accurate AR is 0.76%-0.35%=0.41%. The headline should have read, "Crestor®-Treated Group Had 0.41% Less Heart Attacks as Compared to the Placebo Group." The number-needed-to-treat (NNT) to prevent one heart attack is:

1/0.41%=244

In other words, 244 patients need to be treated with Crestor® for 1.9 years to prevent one heart attack. JUPITER showed that Crestor® failed 99.6% (243/244) since 243 received no benefit in preventing a heart attack. And, at a cost of $2.50/pill, JUPITER showed that it would cost $423,035 to prevent one heart attack– since 244 subjects would need to take the pill daily for 1.9 years to prevent one heart attack[4]. That ridiculous price does not include the price for office visits, laboratory testing and other costs associated with the adverse effects from taking Crestor®.

My analysis clearly shows that JUPITER was a failed study which should have pushed the FDA to consider pulling statins from the marketplace. What happened was the opposite: due to Big Pharma's spin on JUPITER, sales markedly increased.

JUPITER: CRESTOR®-TREATED HAD MORE FATAL HEART ATTACKS

What was not reported in the initial press release was that there were more fatal heart attacks in the Crestor®-treated group as compared to the placebo group. If I were to report this in a RR number, I could state, "The Crestor®-treated group had 43% more fatal heart attacks compared to the placebo group:

$$0.1\%/0.07\% = 1.43$$

Also, what was omitted from the original press release for JUPITER was that the Crestor®-treated group had more diabetes than the control group. Subsequent statin studies have found a significantly increased risk of developing diabetes from statin use. More information about that can be found in Chapter 9.

Due to the initial press releases behind JUPITER, in the third quarter of 2009, sales of Crestor® rose over $1.3 billion as compared with the previous year. Many hailed the findings in

JUPITER as the first study that gave statins the indications for use in primary prevention of heart disease in healthy people.

The JUPITER results were utilized in the newest cholesterol guidelines released in 2013 which dramatically increased the number of people who qualified for taking a statin medication. The new guidelines are discussed in more detail in Chapter 8.

I feel the JUPITER study was another in a long-line of failures for the statinophiles (i.e., those who propose the use of statins for everyone). The positive results with the Crestor®-treated group were miniscule and certainly nothing to set national precedent over. And, that doesn't even include the negative results—more fatal heart attacks and diabetes in the treated group. In fact, this study, like many before and after, should make any health care professional pause when considering whether to ever prescribe a statin or not.

RESULT OF STATIN RANDOMIZED CONTROLLED TRIALS (RCTs) AND MORTALITY

When I was in medical school (1985-1989), I was taught that high cholesterol was a risk factor in heart disease. It was pounded into my head that a lower cholesterol number would lead to a lower risk for heart disease. In fact, it was stated like it was a known fact. That was the basis for the statinophiles to recommend statin drugs for nearly everyone as these drugs are incredibly effective at lowering cholesterol levels. In fact, statinophiles love to check their patients' cholesterol levels and delight in showing their patients that their declining cholesterol levels are due to statins. Furthermore, these health care statinophiles enjoy telling their patients that the falling cholesterol level is good for them as they will suffer less heart attacks and live longer.

Statins are very effective at lowering cholesterol levels. If statinophiles are correct, there has certainly been enough time for statin studies to provide convincing evidence that statins lower the cardiovascular mortality rate in those that take them. However, after more than 20 years, statins have never been shown to significantly lower the cardiovascular mortality rate. I have summarized some of the most important statin studies in Table 5.

As can be seen from Table 5, in every one of the RCTs shown there was no marked decline in mortality when statin users were compared to the control groups. In fact, averaging the 12 studies shows that 764 people would need to be treated for one year to prevent one death. In other words, according to the data from these 12 RCTs, statin drugs failed 99.9% (763/764) in preventing death.

It is clear that the statin studies are nothing worth setting national guidelines by. In fact, the statin studies should give

Table 5 Results of Randomized Controlled Trials of Statins and All-Cause Mortality[5][6][7]

Acronym of RCT	Drug Used	Time (years)	RR (%)	Controls Alive (%)	Treated Alive(%)	AR(%)	AR/Yr (%)	NNT/Yr
Excel	Lovastatin	1	+150	99.7	99.5	+0.3	+0.3	N/A
AFCAPS	Lovastatin	5.2	+3.9	97.7	97.6	+0.1	+0.02	N/A
4S	Simvastatin	5.4	-29	88.5	91.8	-3.3	-0.6	167
HPS	Simvastatin	5	-12	85.3	87.1	-1.8	-0.4	278
WOSCOPS	Pravastatin	4.4	-22	95.9	96.8	-0.9	-0.2	500
PROSPER	Pravastatin	3	-1.9	89.5	89.7	-0.2	-0.1	1429
LIPID	Pravastatin	6.1	-2	85.9	89	-3.1	-0.5	196
CARE	Pravastatin	5	-8	90.6	91.4	-0.8	-0.2	667
ALLHAT	Pravastatin	6	-0.01 ns	87.6	87.8	-0.2	-0.03	3333
FLORIDA	Fluvastatin	1	-35	96.0	97.3	-1.3	-1.3	77
ASCOT	Atorvastatin	3.3	-13	95.9	96.4	-0.5	-0.15	667
JUPITER	Rosuvastatin	1.9	-20	97.2	97.8	-0.6	-0.3	333

the FDA the ammunition it needs to pull them from the marketplace. If statin drugs were free of side effects and inexpensive, then perhaps a case could be made for prescribing millions of people statin drugs. However, statins are neither free of adverse effects nor inexpensive.

WHY DO HEALTH CARE PROFESSIONALS SETTLE FOR SUCH MEDIOCRITY?

Unfortunately, mediocrity is the accepted practice of conventional medicine. I would define mediocrity in medicine as the reason why many, if not most, doctors willingly prescribe expensive medications that have little benefit while at the same time exposing their patients to possible adverse effects.

Why would anyone spend hundreds of millions of advertising dollars trumpeting a 1% success rate in a drug trial? Remember, a 1% success rate means that the drug is a 99% failure as it failed 99% who took it.

The reason that hundreds of millions of dollars were spent after ASCOT is because nearly all health care professionals do not understand statistics. Without a proper understanding of statistics, health care professionals allow The Big Pharma Cartel to pull the wool over their eyes. Big Pharma can tout a 36% effectiveness with a drug when it is truly a 1% success. Furthermore, the lack of understanding of basic statistics allows The Big Pharma Cartel to spew out too-numerous-to-count research articles that show little effect with the most commonly prescribed drugs.   And, keep in mind that these are the studies we see—Big Pharma has failed to release many other negative drug studies.

Years ago, I gave a lecture to a group of conventional cardiologists at a teaching hospital. I presented the ASCOT study as I have presented the data to you. The head of the lipid clinic at the hospital got up in the middle of my presentation and told me, loudly, that I was wrong. I asked him to elaborate. He said that if 1% are helped by the drug, then putting millions on the drug will help a lot of patients. In other words, one million patients treated with Lipitor for 3.3 years could be expected to help 10,000 (since 1% of 1 million is 10,000) avoid a heart attack. However, I pointed out to him that would mean that 990,000 would also have to take Lipitor and would receive no benefit. I further stated that those treated would be exposed to possible side effects and the cost of treating so many patients to help so few is ridiculous. I claimed that prescribing medicines that have a 1% efficacy rate is an example of mediocrity in medicine. Needless to say that did not go over well with the crowd. Since children may read this book, I will not print what was said. At that lecture I felt like I was Alice in Wonderland, where down is up and up is down. But I did come away from that lecture more firmly grounded in my convictions as the cardiologists offered no real arguments refuting my data.

ARE ALL MEDICINES BAD?

That answer is easy: No. Antibiotics to treat bacterial infections such as pneumonia, strep throat and cellulitis are very effective at eradicating the infection. In the case of documented streptococcal throat infection, well over 85% (17 out of 20) are cured of the streptococcal infection with the appropriate antibiotic treatment.[8] Those numbers warrant the use of antibiotics to treat streptococcal infections which prevent serious life-threatening complications. The use of appropriate antibiotics to treat bacterial infections is an example of good medicine as compared to the mediocre use of statins to treat/prevent heart disease.

Final Thoughts

With regard to statistics, medical schools must train their students better. However, it is up to each health care provider to carefully consider whether the drug he/she wants to prescribe will benefit the patient. I am certain that nearly all physicians want to help their patients. However, it is every physician's responsibility to be aware of what the drug does in the body. If he/she is not aware of how the drug works, then it should not be prescribed.

Physicians need to demand more from Big Pharma. None of us, including physicians, would tolerate flying on an airline that failed to get us to our destination 96.5-99% of the time. We would all demand better results. Physicians need to stop prescribing mediocre drugs. Understanding statistics will help physicians make better choices. For those doctors already done with medical school, I suggest re-learning statistics. It will serve you well.

[1] NEJM. Vol 359:2280-2282. 11.20.2008
[2] Am. J. of Med. Vol 118. (12a); 3s-9. 2005
[3] NYT. February 2, 2008
[4] $2.50/pill x 1.9 years x 365 days/year x 244 subjects =$423,035.00.
[5] Adapted from Ravnskov, U. The Cholesterol Myths. 2000. 200-203
[6] Adapted from Kauffman, J. Malignant Medical Myths. 2006. p. 93
[7] Personal communication with Goodman, Ira. Adapted from: The Guide to Anti-Aging and Regenerative Medicine 2013-2018 Edition.
[8] JAMA. 1948;138(14):1030-1036. doi:10.1001/jama.1948.02900140022005

Chapter 8

*Cholesterol Guidelines:
Nonsense Best Avoided*

CHAPTER 8: INTRODUCTION

Every few years, The Powers-That-Be release new cholesterol or dietary guidelines designed to help us avoid the number one killer in the United States—heart disease.

Each time these guidelines are released with fanfare and press coverage. They are promoted in major newspapers and heavily advertised in the print media. If the guidelines were correct from the beginning we would not need new guidelines. I certainly understand that science changes and we need to change our thinking based on scientific studies. However, what does not change is the fact that human biochemistry has been fairly stable over thousands of years. We should be researching and studying items that support and enhance the human biochemical pathways. Unfortunately, most drugs do not support the human biochemical pathways, rather they inhibit them. Recall that the vast majority of drugs work by either poisoning crucial enzymes or blocking important receptors. More information about drug therapies can be found in my book, *Drugs That Don't Work and Natural Therapies That Do.*

This chapter will review the latest guidelines designed to help us prevent coronary artery disease. In 2013, new guidelines about statin use were released by the American College of Cardiology and the American Heart Association.[1] These guidelines were the latest updates designed to help practitioners evaluate, diagnose, and treat those at future risk from heart disease. Before I review the 2013 guidelines, I would like to assess the previous guidelines.

2004 NATIONAL CHOLESTEROL EDUCATION PROGRAM GUIDELINES

The previous set of guidelines for heart disease were updated in 2004 by the National Cholesterol Education Program. The 2004 update called for more intensive cholesterol monitoring and treatment.[2] In fact, the 2004 update commanded that LDL-cholesterol levels should be <70mg/dl in patients at high risk for heart disease. Previously, the guidelines had recommended LDL levels to be <100mg/dl. Keep in mind that it is virtually impossible for the vast majority of adults to have their LDL-cholesterol level <70mg/dl unless they are sick or dying from cancer. My clinical experience has clearly shown that the only way to achieve these numbers is by medicating most (>90%) patients with cholesterol-lowering medications.

The trials used to make these recommendations included:

- Anglo-Scandinavian Cardiac Outcomes Trial Lipid-Lowering Arm (ASCOT-LLA)
- Antihypertensive and Lipid-Lowering Treatment to Prevent Heart Attack Trial Lipid-Lowering Trial (ALLHAT-LLT)
- Heart Protection Study (HPS)
- Prospective Study of Pravastatin in the Elderly at Risk (PROSPER) study

When I was in medical school, I remember rounding with a family doctor—Dr. Barney Solomon. He had a big influence on me in choosing family practice as my specialty. We were rounding on his cardiac patients and I recall asking him how he kept up with all the latest cardiac research. He told me how easy it was. Dr. Solomon said, "David, when you look at a heart study see if there are a lot more people alive at the end of the study. If the drug is saving lives, then it is probably a good one. If more people died, then forget it." I will follow Dr. Solomon's advice and look at the mortality statistics for each of these studies in order to determine if the drug therapy is beneficial or not.

Recall from Chapter 7 on statistics that the absolute risk difference is much more important when deciding whether a particular therapy is valid for a patient. Therefore, I will use the absolute difference in mortality to determine whether the drug therapy was beneficial or not.

1. **Heart Protection Study (HPS)**[3]

The HPS study was performed on 20,536 adults aged 40-80 years. The subjects were randomized to taking Zocor® or placebo for five years. The mortality results showed that the placebo group had 85.4% alive while the Zocor®-treated group had 87.1% alive. The absolute risk reduction (AR) in mortality was **1.7%** (87.1-85.4).

2. **Prospective Study of Pravastatin in the Elderly at Risk (PROSPER)**[4]

PROSPER enrolled 5,804 adults to take either Pravachol® or placebo for three years. At the end of the study, the mortality results showed that the placebo group had 89.5% alive while the Pravachol® group had 89.7% alive. The absolute risk reduction (AR) in mortality declined **0.2%**.

3. **Antihypertensive and Lipid-Lowering Treatment to Prevent Heart Attack Trial Lipid-Lowering Trial (ALLHAT-LLT)**[5]

ALLHAT encompassed 10,355 adults over 55 years old to

take either Pravachol® or placebo for eight years. At the end of the study, 84.7% of the placebo group was alive versus 85.1% of the treated group. The absolute risk reduction (AR) in mortality difference was **0.4%,** which was non-significant.

4. **Anglo-Scandinavian Cardiac Outcomes Trial Lipid-Lowering Arm (ASCOT-LLA)**[6]

ASCOT was reviewed in more detail in Chapter 7. This study enrolled 19,342 hypertensive subjects between the ages of 40-79. They were randomized to a control group and a placebo group treated with Lipitor®. After 3.3 years, 95.9% of the control group was alive versus 96.4% of the Lipitor®-treated group. The absolute risk reduction (AR) in mortality was **0.465%** in the Lipitor®-treated group.

SUMMARY OF THE FOUR STUDIES

The summary of these four "evidence-based" studies (shown in Table 1) showed no dramatic difference in mortality between those that took a statin and those that took a placebo. In fact, in the four studies, there was a measly 0.775% absolute mortality decline in those that used a statin when compared to those that used a placebo. A 0.775% decline can also be written as 0.00775.

In other words, according to the data from the four studies that used a placebo, 129 patients would need to take a statin for

Table 1: Summary of Four Studies

Study	Drug	Length (yrs)	Placebo Group Alive	Treatment Group Alive	Absolute Risk Reduction (AR) in Mortality
HPS	Zocor®	5	85.4%	87.1%	1.7%
PROSPER	Pravachol®	3	89.5%	89.7%	0.2%
ALLHAT-LLT	Pravachol	8	84.7%	85.1%	0.4%
ASCOT-LLA	Lipitor	3.3	95.9%	96.4%	0.5%

approximately five years (the average length of the studies) to prevent one death. As I stated in Chapter 7, this is known as the number-needed-to-treat. It is a statistical number that helps health care professionals decide whether a particular therapy is beneficial or not.

Let's assume that Lipitor® costs $135/month. (A call to a local pharmacy confirmed that amount). Therefore, to prevent one death, these four studies estimated that it would cost $1,044,900.00 ($135 patient cost/month x 12 months/year x 5 years x 129 patients).

Is $1,044,900.00 an acceptable amount to prevent one death? Perhaps the answer could be yes if the drug was not associated with adverse effects for the 99% (128/129) who received no benefit. However, Chapter 9 will show you that statins are, in fact, associated with many serious side effects. Furthermore, the high number-needed-to-treat provides compelling evidence that statins are not effective at improving mortality numbers in the vast majority who take them.

THE 2013 AMERICAN COLLEGE OF CARDIOLOGY/AMERICAN HEART ASSOCIATION (ACC/AHA) TREATMENT OF BLOOD CHOLESTEROL TO REDUCE ATHEROSCLEROTIC CARDIOVASCULAR RISK IN ADULTS

When the 2013 ACC/AHA Guidelines were published, the new guidelines were met with much fanfare.[7] There were articles in many newspapers and magazines touting the new guidelines as the best way to prevent heart disease. In fact, the American Heart Association stated, "The new cardiovascular prevention guidelines were written based on years of scientific research to develop the best approaches to preventing heart disease and stroke–the leading causes of death in the world."[8]

The 2013 ACC/AHA Guidelines recommend statins in four groups (if your risk of developing cardiac disease is greater than 7.5% over a ten-year period):

1. Adults with clinical atherosclerotic coronary vascular disease
2. Adults with LDL-Cholesterol >190mg/dl

3. Adults 40-75 years of age with diabetes
4. Adults >7.5% estimated 10-year risk of atherosclerotic coronary vascular disease

I will provide my opinion on treating each of these four groups of people with statins later in this chapter.

Unlike previous guidelines, there are no total cholesterol treatment targets. Finally, The Powers-That-Be agree that following cholesterol numbers is useless. Well, sort of. Although there are no target cholesterol levels, the total cholesterol and HDL-cholesterol levels are still used to determine one's heart disease risk factor.

Furthermore, the 2013 Guidelines have, for the first time, recommended statin therapy for primary prevention—for use in those individuals who have not had a cardiac event and are trying to prevent the first one.

The 2013 Guidelines markedly increase the number of Americans who would qualify for taking a statin. Based on the National Health and Nutrition Examination Survey (NHANES), 50% of all African-American men and 30% of Caucasian men in their 50's would now qualify for a statin medication. By age 70, the new guidelines would recommend nearly all men take a statin medication. For women, the new guidelines would place 70% of African American women and 60% of Caucasian women in their 60's on statin medications.

Challenges to the 2013 ACC/AHA Guidelines to Reduce Coronary Artery Disease

I feel the 2013 ACC/AHA Guidelines widely overstated the benefits of statin medications, particularly in primary prevention, and understated, or worse, ignored, the adverse effects of statin medications.

As previously stated, If your risk of developing cardiac disease is greater than 7.5% over a ten year period, then statins are recommended. The risk can be calculated by going to the American Heart Association website (www.heart.org) and plugging in your cholesterol and HDL-cholesterol numbers as well as your age and whether you smoke or not. Then a number is revealed.

It is hard for me to believe that this simple numerical formula is what modern medicine has come to. When you think about it, it is rather pathetic. I guess nobody needs to see a health care professional anymore—just put your numbers in and if you have a 10-year heart attack risk of >7.5%, then you must take a statin for the rest of your life. I have one word for this nonsense: "Fugetaboutit."

The new guidelines are contained in an 85 page, mind-numbing document. It is a very difficult manuscript to read. I will dissect parts of it for you.

Let's start with the recommendations that would put most adult Americans on statin drugs. On page 18, the report states, "Data has shown that statins used for primary prevention have substantial ASCVD (atherosclerotic cardiovascular disease) risk reduction benefits across the range of LDL–C levels of 70-189 mg/dL." Of course, that is after the "experts" state that it is unclear if lowering LDL-cholesterol levels have any benefit. Nonetheless, the authors cite a meta-analysis by the Cholesterol Treatment Trialists' (CTT) to support their conclusion.[9]

The CTT study was a meta-analysis of 27 randomized trials to ascertain whether reducing LDL-cholesterol levels with statin use reduces vascular events in people who are at a low-risk for cardiac events. The authors of the article reported that reduction in LDL-cholesterol levels with a statin reduced the risk of major vascular events by 21%. However, this is a relative risk reduction (RR). When deciding whether to prescribe a statin for a patient, the 21% relative risk reduction should not be used. Remember, I reviewed the inaccuracy and the problems associated with using the relative risk in medical studies. The relative risk is pushed by Big Pharma because it overstates the benefits of mediocre pharmaceuticals. Unfortunately, most (or nearly all) doctors have virtually no understanding about statistics and what relative risk means. As I previously stated, physicians should not be prescribing medications if they cannot understand the statistical research in the studies used to promote the drugs.

As previously stated, the absolute risk reduction has more clinical meaning than the relative risk. In fact, a clinical decision on whether to prescribe a drug or not should not be based on the relative risk numbers, rather it should be based on the absolute risk data. The absolute risk reduction of cardiovascular disease in the CTT study was 0.77%. The authors should have reported, "The reduction in LDL-cholesterol levels with a statin reduced the risk of major vascular events by 0.77%." Therefore, according to the CTT numbers, 130 people would need to be treated with a statin for at least five years (the average length of the studies) to prevent one vascular event. That means that 129 subjects took the statin without any benefit and they could have developed adverse effects. In other words, this study showed that statins failed 99.2% of those (129/130) who took them.

So, tell me, does this study make you want to take a statin to prevent a vascular event? If anything, it should make you think the opposite. It is amazing to think that The Powers-That-Be set clinical guidelines on such an underwhelming study. If anything, the CTT study is another nail-in-the-coffin showing statin medications fail the vast majority who take them.

Once someone has a diagnosis of heart disease, if they are prescribed a statin medication, they would be taking it for secondary prevention. That means, they have already suffered a cardiac event and are trying to prevent a new one.

Most of the statin studies have been done with patients who have already suffered a cardiac event. The best of the secondary prevention studies show a 1-3.5% reduction in death from heart attacks after taking a statin for 3-5 years (the average length of the studies). That means that 96.5-99% of people who have already suffered a cardiac event are not helped by taking a statin medication.

CHALLENGES TO THE ACC/AHA 2013 GUIDELINES

1. Adults with Clinical Atherosclerotic Coronary Vascular Disease

This recommendation has to do with the secondary prevention of coronary vascular disease. Remember, a secondary prevention recommendation means the patient has already suffered a cardiac event and the new recommendation is designed to prevent further cardiac events.

As I showed you in Chapter 7, the best of the statin studies for secondary prevention of cardiac illness show a 1-3.5% (AR) reduced risk of heart attacks or mortality from taking a statin drug if it is used for a minimum of 3-5 years (the length of most statin studies). That means the drugs failed 96.5-99% of those who took them as they received no mortality or heart attack benefit.

Adults do not get atherosclerotic coronary vascular disease because of a lack of statin medications. They have heart disease because they are suffering from excess inflammation due to infections, eating a poor diet, nutritional and hormonal imbalances, heavy metal toxicity, etc. These items will be covered in future chapters. And, each of these factors cause the body to increase its production of cholesterol and LDL in order to counteract these issues.

2. Adults with LDL-Cholesterol >190mg/dl

With the way that conventional doctors rail about LDL-cholesterol, you would think it must be a very dangerous substance.

However, I established in Chapter 3 that LDL-cholesterol is not a dangerous substance. In fact, it is a crucial molecule needed by the body not only to shuttle cholesterol around but also to fight infections. Furthermore, It also functions as an anti-inflammatory agent.

Cholesterol, an essential molecule for every cell in the body, must be transported to the tissues by LDL lipoproteins (named LDL-cholesterol). LDL-cholesterol carries cholesterol from the liver to the tissues.

There are studies that correlate high LDL-cholesterol levels with an increased risk of heart disease. There are others that fail to show the correlation. However, LDL is not the problem, rather it is just doing what the body is asking of it; shuttling cholesterol from the liver to the tissues and helping fight infections and acting as an anti-inflammatory agent.

For example, people who lose weight lower their cholesterol and LDL-cholesterol level.[10] Cardiologists would seize upon the lowered LDL-cholesterol levels and claim, "This is good. Your lowered LDL-cholesterol level has lowered your risk of heart disease."

However, I would state, the lowered risk of heart disease is not from the lowered LDL-cholesterol level, but rather from the weight loss. LDL-cholesterol is just the bystander here. The analogy I will repeat is that blaming LDL-cholesterol levels for causing heart disease is similar to blaming firemen for causing fires since firemen are present at all fires.

In the case of an obese patient, they will need elevated cholesterol levels to combat the inflammation that is occurring due to the excess inflammatory-provoking tissue—fat stores. In this case, the body is doing exactly what it should be doing—delivering more cholesterol to the tissues to try and protect it from the inflammatory fires that are burning. The best treatment for this case is to lose weight as this will naturally lower cholesterol and LDL-cholesterol levels. Chemically blocking LDL production will not result in a long-term beneficial effect.

More about LDL-cholesterol can be found in Chapter 3.

3. Adults 40-75 years of age with diabetes

I find it beyond ridiculous that most adults with diabetes are now recommended to be placed on a statin medication.

Why is this ridiculous?

It is ridiculous because statins have been shown to increase the risk for developing diabetes.

Now, there are a large number of studies pointing out that statins significantly increase the risk for diabetes and the risk increases the longer you take a statin medication. Statins may increase this risk by impairing pancreatic beta cell function (where insulin is produced) and decreasing insulin sensitivity. The JUPITER trial clearly showed a significant increased risk of diabetes with statin therapy after 1.9 years of statin therapy (with Crestor®).[11]

I find it interesting that new statin guidelines recommend treating a diabetic with statins. Perhaps the new guidelines are trying to make new patients! (That last sentence was said tongue-in-cheek. Sort of.)

4. Adults >7.5% estimated 10-year risk of atherosclerotic coronary vascular disease

People can figure out their risk by using an online calculator found at www. heart.org.

The 10-year risk calculator for atherosclerotic coronary vascular disease was rolled out with great fanfare when the 2013 ACC/AHA Guidelines were released. Shortly afterwards, there were critical articles written about it.[12] Estimates were that the calculator over-estimated risk in certain groups by over 50%.

Why is a 7.5% risk the cutoff that determines who takes a statin or not? That has never been explained. Another question is why would The Powers-That-Be release a risk calculator that over-estimated the risk for heart disease? The answer is simple; over-estimating the risk provided millions of more patients for Big Pharma to treat with statins. When the calculator was exposed as a fraud, the guideline authors offered a feeble defense. They stated that the guidelines were never intended to be taken at face value.[13]

I say a better response should have been to get rid of the calculator from the start. As for the calculator: Again I say, "Fugetaboutit."

LIFESTYLE MODIFICATIONS AND THE 2013 GUIDELINES

The 2013 Guidelines also acknowledge the importance of lifestyle modifications. The authors state that lifestyle modifications should include eating a diet high in fruits, vegetables, fish, and low in sweets, red meat, and sodium. Furthermore, the Guidelines state that regular moderate to vigorous physical activity is recommended to prevent heart disease.

They got some of the lifestyle modifications correct— eating a diet high in fruits and vegetables, fish, and low in sweets. And, they correctly recommended exercise.

However, they erred in suggesting a low sodium diet. Salt is the second major constituent in the body next to water. The human body needs and requires adequate amounts of salt to function optimally. In fact, a low-salt diet has been shown to cause an increased risk of heart attacks, an increase in insulin levels and an increase in lipid levels which include both cholesterol and LDL-cholesterol levels. In other words, low-salt diets cause heart disease. Chapter 14 will discuss the importance of salt as it relates to heart disease. And, more information on the health benefits of salt can be found in my book, *Salt Your Way to Health*.

Final Thoughts

The 2013 American College of Cardiology/American Heart Association (ACC/AHA) Treatment of Blood Cholesterol to Reduce Atherosclerotic Cardiovascular Risk in Adults should be placed with the earlier guidelines: in the dustpan.

Until conventional medicine truly searches for the underlying cause of heart disease, we are stuck with ridiculous cholesterol guidelines and poor drug therapies that do not address the underlying issues. Statin medications are ineffective for the vast majority who take them. They neither reduced heart attack nor mortality rates significantly. Furthermore, their side-effect profile is unacceptable.

Heart disease is not killing a majority of our population because they are suffering from a statin-deficiency syndrome. Rather, people are developing heart disease from smoking, nutritional deficiencies, infections, and eating a poor diet. Addressing these issues will be more productive than reflexively treating everyone with a statin medication.

[1] J. of Am. College of Card. 2014. Vol. 63, N. 25.
[2] Circulation 2004; 110:227-239
[3] Lancet 2002;360:7-22
[4] Lancet. 2002;360:1623-1630
[5] JAMA *2002; 288: 2998-3007*
[6] AJM. 2005. V. 118(12a), 3s-9s
[7] JACC Vol. 63, No. 25, 2014
[8] Accessed 1.9.15 from: http://www.heart.org/HEARTORG/General/What-Guidelines-Mean-To-You-Infographic_UCM_459169_SubHomePage.jsp

[9] Lancet. 2012;380;581-90

[10] Am. J. of Cardiology. 59,9G-17G. 1987
[11] N Engl J Med 2008;359: 2195–207
[12] JAMA Intern. Med. doi:10.1001/jamainternmed.2014.5336
[13] JAMA Intern. Med. IBID. 2014.

Chapter 9

Adverse Effects of Statins

CHAPTER 9: INTRODUCTION

As I showed you in Chapter 8, the most recent (2013) American College of Cardiology/American Heart Association (ACC/AHA) Guidelines markedly increased the number of Americans for whom a statin medication would be recommended. The new guidelines introduced a prediction model for cardiovascular disease and lowered the threshold for treatment with statins to a 7.5% ten-year risk.[1] Health care providers were instructed to use a risk calculator to determine a patient's risk of developing cardiovascular disease over the following ten years. However, the risk calculator was shown to be flawed as it overestimated the risk of cardiovascular disease. "The poor performance of the risk calculator is self-evident to any clinician who attempts to make a calculation for {a patient}."[2]

However, not all physicians believe that following the ACC/AHA guidelines would overestimate the numbers of patients who should be taking a statin medication. In fact, a recent study found nearly 100% of men and 62% of women aged 66 to 75 should take a statin medication even if their cholesterol level is normal.[3]

This chapter will be devoted to the adverse drug reactions that have been associated with statins. This chapter could not have been written without the work of Philip Blair, M.D. Dr. Blair was able to collate the FDA data about adverse effects from statins using the FDA Adverse Events Databases.[4]

ADVERSE DRUG REACTIONS

In my book, *Drugs That Don't Work and Natural Therapies That Do*, I describe how most prescription medications work in the human body. In fact, nearly all prescription medications work by poisoning enzymes or blocking receptors in the body. In this book, I state, "You can't poison a crucial enzyme or block an important receptor for the long-term and expect a good result."

An adverse drug reaction is any noxious, unintended or undesired effect of a drug that was appropriately used. In other words, the drug was taken and prescribed appropriately, yet an untoward effect occurred due to the use of the drug.

In 1994, researchers studied six major medical centers in the U.S. and recorded how many adverse reactions occurred in hospitalized patients. Also, these same scientists calculated the number of hospitalized patients who died from an adverse drug reaction. From these numbers, the scientists extrapolated how many adverse drug reactions occurred throughout the U.S. in hospitalized patients. They reported that in 1994, over 2.2 million adverse drug reactions resulted in over 106,000 deaths.[5] This number of deaths—106,000—is similar to a jumbo jet full of patients dying every day in U.S. hospitals, not from their illness but rather from taking a medication that was appropriately prescribed and given to them. You are probably asking yourself, "How can this occur?"

As I have previously stated, the reason that there are so many adverse drug reactions is that nearly all medications work by poisoning enzymes or blocking receptors in the body. It is my premise that the human body was not designed to have its receptors blocked or its enzymes poisoned. In fact, when a drug is found to block receptors or poison enzymes, a keen mind (or even a feeble mind) should be able to predict that the drug will be associated with adverse reactions.

Keep in mind, the adverse drug reaction study I quoted above was completed in 1994. Over 20 years later, we are using many more prescription medications that work the same way as the previous ones did; they block receptors and/or poison enzymes in the body. There is no doubt that as we take more medications we will be prone to suffer more adverse drug reactions.

This is not to say that all drugs that poison enzymes and block receptors are bad drugs. There are times to use medications that work this way such as in the middle of an acute heart attack. However, for the long-term treatment of a medical problem, it is generally unwise to rely on drugs that poison enzymes or block receptors. Americans take more prescription drugs that any people have ever taken, yet we suffer from worse outcomes on nearly every health indicator that has ever been studied.

WHY DO MOST DRUGS POISON ENZYMES AND BLOCK RECEPTORS?

That is another million dollar question. The answer to this one is easy: The Big Pharma Cartel can only patent synthetic agents; they cannot patent a natural item. For example, vitamins C, D, and E cannot be patented as they are natural substances. However, statins, being a foreign substance to the body, can be patented.

Big Pharma's goal is to patent a substance. Therefore, it can hold the rights to the item and profits will be maximized. If

Big Pharma discovered a natural product that cured heart disease, then anyone could manufacture it after the reports of a cure are released. Now you can see why Big Pharma has no interest in using natural products.

The human body has receptors for natural substances. It also has mechanisms—detoxification pathways—useful for removing these items when the body is done with them.

However, the same is not true for synthetic items. The human body has no receptors for most synthetic items and it does not have efficient detoxification methods to remove them. That is why the half-life for most drugs is very long when it is compared to a natural item. The half-life of a drug refers to how long it takes for 50% of the drug to be cleared from the body. For example, the hormone progesterone has a half-life of twenty minutes. The half-life of Depo-Provera, the synthetic form of progesterone, is 50 days. It is no wonder that Depo-Provera is associated with a host of adverse effects including invasive breast cancer, blood clots, pulmonary edema and irreversible osteoporosis. Natural, bioidentical progesterone has no such adverse effects. More about this can be found in my book, *The Miracle of Natural Hormones*.

Natural substances generally have shorter half-lives when compared to synthetic items. That is because the body has receptors and knows what to do with the substance. It can easily be predicted that a longer half-life of a drug will result in an increase of adverse effects. Keep in mind that most natural substances have a half-life of minutes to a few hours. The half-life of Lipitor is 20-30 hours.[6] The half-life of Crestor is 19 hours.[7] It is also important to note that a drug's half-life is markedly increased in the elderly as their renal and hepatic functions decline with aging.

STATINS AND ADVERSE DRUG REACTIONS

Chapter 6 reviewed the mechanism of the action of statin medications. Recall that statin medications work by poisoning the enzyme HMG-CoA reductase.

Statins are associated with a wide range of adverse reactions. This could be predicted if one knows that cholesterol is such an important molecule for each and every cell in the body. In fact, every organ system could be predicted to be adversely impacted by a statin medication. Any percentage increase in adverse effects reported in this chapter are referred to as relative risk numbers unless otherwise indicated.

Figure 1 lists some of the adverse effects of statins. The remainder of this section will discuss some of these adverse effects. I will also list the reports made to the Food and Drug Administration Adverse Event Reporting System (FAERS). The data from FAERS was compiled by my fellow THINCS (The

Figure 1: Adverse Effects of Statins

ALS or ALS-like syndrome	Lupus
Aneurysm	Macular degeneration
Atrial fibrillation	Memory loss
Autoimmune illness	Myalgia
Bell's Palsy	Myopathy
Breast Cancer	Myositis
Cancer	Neuropathy
Cataracts	New difficulty walking
CoQ10 depletion	Oroantral fistula
Dementia	Pancreatitis
Depression	Parkinson's disease
Diabetes	Peripheral neuropathy
Exercise limitations	Prostate Cancer
Guillain-Barre	Rhabdomyolysis
Gynecomastia	Renal Insufficiency
Heart failure	Rippling muscle disease
Hepatic dysfunction	Sexual dysfunction
Hepatitis B reactivation	Serotonin receptor depletion
Hyperkalemia	Skin cancer
Hypertension	Spermatozoa dysfunction
Increased risk of infection	Sleep difficulties
Inflammatory myopathies	Tendinopathy
Irritability/aggression	Testosterone deficiency
Kidney damage	Thyroid disorders
Liver pathology	Weight gain

International Network of Cholesterol Skeptics) friend and colleague, Philip W. Blair, M.D.

The adverse drug reaction most commonly associated with a statin medication occurs in the muscles. The reason statins can cause muscle problems is due, in part, to the depletion of Coenzyme Q10 (CoQ10). CoQ10 is a vitamin-like substance produced in the mitochondria of the body. The highest concentration of CoQ10 occurs in the muscles, particularly the heart muscle. It is needed to produce ATP, the energy storage molecule. In fact, over 90% of the body's energy is produced using CoQ10 as a cofactor.[8] Any process which results in a depletion of CoQ10 could be expected to result in energy and muscle issues. Two of the most common adverse effects of statins are fatigue and muscle aches and pains.

MUSCLE DAMAGE, CoQ10, AND STATINS

However, there are many more muscle adverse effects that occur from statins. During the same ten-year span, there were 44,838 reports to the FDA of muscle complaints caused by statins including pain, stiffness, weakness, cramps, fatigue, and myalgia (muscle pain). They can be broken down further:

- Musculoskeletal stiffness and tightness: 3,427 reports
- Muscle cramps: 537 reports
- Myalgia: 18,416 reports

The heart is the largest muscle in the body. It also has the largest concentration of CoQ10 in the body. From 2004-2014, there were 40,476 cases of heart issues related to statins reported to the FDA. This includes 19,831 heart attacks and 12,305 heart failure adverse event reports due to statin use.

None of these numbers should be surprising once you understand that CoQ10, which is inhibited by statins, is necessary for proper heart muscle functioning. In fact, congestive heart failure is increasing at epidemic rates. I have no doubt that it is increasing so rapidly because of the widespread use of statin medications.

Why Would A Drug Which Poisons The Enzyme That Is Needed to Make CoQ10 Be Prescribed?

CoQ10 is mostly found in the mitochondria—the energy powerhouse of the cells. CoQ10 is part of oxidative phosphorylation where the energy storage molecule ATP is produced.

CoQ10 has other functions as well. It is a strong antioxidant which has been shown to protect mitochondrial DNA from oxidation. CoQ10 works with many substances in the body including vitamins B2 and B3, as well as vitamins C and E. CoQ10 is an integral substance that muscle cells use to produce energy so that the muscles can optimally perform. Inadequate CoQ10 levels are associated with muscle problems such as heart disease, congestive heart failure and other myopathies.

CoQ10 supplementation may help a patient suffering with statin-associated myalgia. My experience has shown that the addition of CoQ10 to a patient who is suffering with statin-associated myalgia will have variable effects; some will be helped, others will not improve. More will improve simply by stopping the statin medication. In fact, every patient suffering from statin-associated myalgia should stop the statin medication.

A trial of 32 subjects with hypercholesterolemia and statin-associated myopathy were randomized to take CoQ10 or vitamin E along with a statin. Compared to the vitamin E group, the CoQ10 group showed a 40% decrease in pain and a 38% reduction in pain interference with daily activities.[9]

Forty-four patients with statin-associated myopathy were randomly assigned to take 200mg/day of CoQ10 or placebo for twelve weeks all the while titrating the statin dose upward. At the end of the study, CoQ10 levels increased in the treatment group but the muscle-pain scores failed to change.[10]

Many physicians are under the mistaken impression that taking CoQ10 supplementation along with a statin will mitigate the myalgia adverse effects. CoQ10 will be inhibited with the use of statins. There is no doubt about that statement. In fact, research has shown that statins can reduce CoQ10 levels by nearly 50%.[11]

However, it is not that simple. In fact, many studies have shown that CoQ10 supplementation will not protect against or reverse statin-associated myopathy. Researchers studied 49 patients with high cholesterol levels who were randomly assigned to CoQ10 or placebo in combination with a statin medication for 16 weeks. The CoQ10 levels increased in the treatment group and decreased in the placebo group, but muscle injury markers did not differ between the two groups.[12]

Congestive Heart Failure, CoQ10 and Statins

Congestive heart failure (CHF) occurs when the heart muscle weakens. As a result of a weakened heart muscle, the heart cannot pump enough blood and oxygen to the organs and tissues of the body. As CHF worsens, fluid begins to build up in the lungs and the extremities.

Unfortunately, CHF is common. CHF is the third most common cause of cardiovascular disease in the U.S.[13] Approximately 5.1 million people in the U.S. have congestive heart failure.[14] It is estimated that one in nine deaths in the U.S.

is due to CHF.[15] CHF is estimated to cost the U.S. over $32 billion per year.[16] Over 550,000 new cases of CHF are diagnosed each year in the U.S. The risk for developing CHF increases as the age increases. In fact, CHF affects 1% of those over 50 years. For those over 75 years, 5% have CHF and over 25% of those greater than 85 years suffer with CHF.

However, the most telling statistic related to CHF is that 50% of those diagnosed with heart failure will die within five years of that diagnosis.

Congestive heart failure can be caused from high blood pressure, diabetes, and coronary heart disease. It is also increased in cigarette smokers and in those suffering from obesity.

However, the most overlooked cause of congestive heart failure is statin use resulting in CoQ10 deficiency. Clinical studies of CoQ10 and CHF date back over 35 years.[17] As previously stated, CoQ10 is primarily found in the mitochondria in muscle tissue. The highest concentration of CoQ10 in the body is in the heart—the largest muscle in the body. Studies have shown that plasma CoQ10 concentration was an independent predictor of mortality in patients with CHF.[18]

Recall that CoQ10 is produced in the same pathway that

produces cholesterol. CoQ10 is produced down-stream from cholesterol—see Figure 1 page 92. Therefore, statins, by inhibiting the enzyme HMG-CoA reductase, will result in a lowered production of CoQ10.

In CHF, the weakness of the heart is manifested as poor contractility. This can be measured as the heart ejection fraction—in other words, what percent of the blood in the heart is the heart able to pump out to the body. A recent study found CoQ10 supplementation, as compared to a placebo group, significantly improved the ejection fraction in patients with CHF by 3.7%.[19]

All congestive heart failure patients should have a therapeutic trial of CoQ10—about 300mg/day. It has been reported that serum CoQ10 concentrations should be greater than 2µg/ml to improve the ejection fraction in CHF.[20]

RHABDOMYOLYSIS AND STATINS

One of the most serious adverse drug reactions due to a statin medication is a condition called rhabdomyolysis. Rhabdomyolysis is a condition where damaged skeletal muscle tissue breaks down. The breakdown products include the muscle protein myoglobin. Myoglobin is an iron and oxygen binding protein that is only found in the blood stream after muscle injury. Myoglobin released into the blood stream must be cleared by the kidneys. However, the kidneys can become damaged when they are exposed to myoglobin. Kidney failure can be caused from myoglobin exposure. Rhabdomyolysis can be a life-threatening condition.

Rhabdomyolysis can be caused by excess physical exercise, a crush injury, a blood clot that disrupts blood flow to the muscle, and by statin use. Baycol®, an older statin medication, was withdrawn from the market in 2001 after there were numerous reports of rhabdomyolysis associated with it. Although most doctors think that the risk of statins causing rhabdomyolysis is very low, thousands of cases of rhabdomyolysis have been reported to the FDA.

In fact, over a 10-year period (2004-2014), there were 10,388 cases of rhabdomyolysis reported to the FDA.

Statins and Exercise

Statins can injure muscle cells. Sometimes this is reflected in blood tests that monitor for muscle enzymes. However, many times statin-treated patients suffer with myalgias without abnormal laboratory tests.

Many physicians feel that if the laboratory tests fail to show elevated muscle enzymes then the statin medication is not responsible for the muscle pains. This thinking is wrong.

Researchers studied four groups to determine if muscle pain reflects muscle injury in the form of elevated muscle enzymes:[21]

- Control Group (no statin use)
- Former statin user with muscle pain (average of 12 weeks off a statin medication)
- Current statin users with myopathy
- Current statin users without myopathy

A muscle biopsy was performed in all the subjects. Each muscle biopsy was evaluated under a microscope to look for signs of muscle damage. The researchers visualized muscle injury in 25 (of 44) patients with myopathy and in one patient without myopathy. Only one patient with structural injury had elevated muscle enzyme levels. The authors concluded, "A lack of elevated levels of {muscle enzymes} does not rule out structural muscle injury."

This study also showed that 60% of former statin users— off statins for an average of 12 weeks—had damaged muscle fibers when the biopsy was evaluated by microscopy. And, 5% of current statin users without muscle complaints exhibited damaged muscle fibers under microscopy.

This is a very important study because few statin users have their muscles biopsied to ascertain the health of their muscle fibers. It is beyond belief that 60% of former statin users—off statins for an average of 12 weeks—can still be exhibiting signs of muscle damage under microscopy. Any medication that damages the tissue after it has been removed for 12 weeks should be pulled from the marketplace. Can you imagine how quickly the Food and Drug Administration (FDA) would pull a natural substance that was reported to damage muscle fibers 12 weeks after the patient stopped taking it?

Statins and the Brain

The highest concentration of cholesterol in the body occurs in the brain, particularly the cortex or the thinking part of the brain. Knowing this, one can easily predict that taking a statin medication, since it is effective in lowering cholesterol, will cause an increased risk for brain problems.

STATINS AND ADVERSE EFFECTS TO THE BRAIN

From 2004-2014, reports to the FDA found that statins caused:

- Amnesia: 4,720 cases
- Confusional State: 7,171 cases
- Dementia: 1,577 cases
- Disorientation: 2,054 cases
- Depression: 13,290 cases

- Memory impairment and transient global amnesia: 9,044 cases
- Suicidal ideation, attempt, or behavior: 3,414 cases

STATINS AND TRANSIENT GLOBAL AMNESIA

Transient global amnesia is the sudden, temporary episode of memory loss. It is characterized by a vanishing of all recent events where one cannot remember where they are or how they got there. My THINCS colleague and friend, Duanne Graveline, M.D. has written extensively about statins. Dr. Graveline is known as 'Spacedoc" as he was a NASA physician. Dr. Graveline had his own personal experience with taking a statin drug. The following story is excerpted from his book, "*The Statin Damage Crisis*."[22]

"My personal introduction to the incredible world of TGA--{transient global amnesia} occurred six weeks after Lipitor® was started during my annual astronaut physical at Johnson Space Center. My cholesterol had been trending upward for several years and all was well until six weeks later when my wife found me aimlessly walking about the yard after my usual walk in the woods. I did not recognize her, reluctantly accepted cookies and milk and refused to go into my now unfamiliar home. I awoke six hours later in the office of my examining neurologist with the diagnosis of transient global amnesia, cause unknown. My MRI several days later was normal. Since Lipitor® was the only new

medicine I was on, the doctor in me made me suspect a possible side effect of this drug and, despite the protestations of the examining doctors that statin drugs did not do this, I stopped my Lipitor®.

The year passed uneventfully and soon it was time for my next astronaut physical. NASA doctors joined the chorus...that statin drugs did not do this and at their bidding I reluctantly restarted Lipitor® at one-half the previous dose. Six weeks later I again descended into the black pit of amnesia, this time for twelve hours and with a retrograde loss of memory back to my high school days. During this terrible interval, when my entire adult life had been eradicated, I had no awareness of my marriage, and children, my medical school days, my ten adventure-filled years as a USAF flight surgeon or my selection as NASA scientist astronaut. All had vanished from my mind as completely as if they had never happened. Fortunately, my memory returned spontaneously..."

Dr. Graveline's case is not unique. The medical literature reports many case histories of statin-associated amnesia. As stated above, there have been 9,044 cases of amnesia related to statin use reported to the FDA over a 10-year period.

It is not just transient amnesic episodes that should worry statin users. Statins may negatively affect the brain function in 100% who take them. Researchers have correlated cognitive impairment in 100% of statin users if the appropriate testing is done.[23]

Statins have been associated with depression and cognitive decline. This could be predicted as the highest concentration of cholesterol occurs in the brain.

A search of PubMed revealed 282 articles about statins and depression. To be fair, there are some studies that show statins are associated with a decreased rate of depression.[24] However, knowing that the brain has the highest concentration of cholesterol would lead one to predict that chemically lowering cholesterol levels would be associated with adverse brain effects such as depression and cognitive decline.

A study of 329 elderly (>65 years) subjects compared mental status tests between statin users and non-users of statins. Statin users were found to have lower mental status scores and higher depressive scores.[25] The authors summarized their findings by stating there are "...substantial indications that caution should be exercised in the provision of statins in elderly subjects to avoid accelerated memory loss."

A recent study found the use of statins after a stroke was associated with a 65% increased risk of depression when compared to stroke survivors who did not take a statin.[26]

My clinical experience has shown that statin use is associated with an increase in depressive symptoms as well as a decline in cognitive functioning.

Neuropathy and Statins

From 2004-2014, FAERS reports to the FDA have found that statins have been reported to cause:

- 5,950 cases of neuropathy
- 15,580 cases of pain in the extremities
- 3,742 cases of balance disorders
- 736 cases of coordination problems

Neuropathy is a very painful condition characterized by pain, fine muscle twitching, muscle loss, change in balance and coordination, numbness, and tingling. Furthermore, neuropathy can manifest as hypertension, arrhythmias, or bone degeneration. The most common manifestation of neuropathy is pain and tingling of the extremities—this is known as peripheral neuropathy.

Neuropathy can have many causes including trauma and diabetes. Statins are well-known to be an underlying cause of neuropathy.

STATINS AND MYELIN

Myelin is the substance that covers the outside of the

nerves—known as the myelin sheath. It acts like an insulator that protects the nerves. It is an essential substance that is produced by the glial cells of the nervous system.

Cholesterol is the main constituent of myelin. In the mature brain, the highest concentration of cholesterol is found in the myelin.[27] Brain maturation and metabolism depends on adequate myelin levels. Myelin is also necessary for nerve fibers to regenerate when they are damaged. A damaged nerve fiber needs the myelin sheath to provide a tract for the nerve to regrow.

Demyelination refers to the loss of the myelin sheath and is associated with some neurodegenerative disorders such as multiple sclerosis, Guillain-Barre syndrome and demyelinating polyneuropathy.

From 2004-2014, FAERS reports to the FDA have found that statins have been reported to cause:

- 202 cases of Guillain-Barre syndrome
- 334 cases of amyotrophic lateral sclerosis (ALS or Lou Gehrig's disease)
- 1,330 cases of multiple sclerosis

When you understand that the myelin sheath is primarily made from cholesterol, it is not a leap of faith to assume that chemically disrupting cholesterol production will cause demyelination conditions. That is exactly what is happening as shown in the literature. One study found statin use associated with a 270% increased risk of idiopathic (unknown cause) polyneuropathy. For patients treated with statins for two or more years, there was a 26.4x increased risk of polyneuropathy.[28] The authors concluded, "We found that users of statins were at a 4- to 14-fold increased risk of developing idiopathic polyneuropathy compared with the background population, and that this adverse effect may primarily occur after long-term treatment with statins. Long-term exposure to statins may substantially increase the risk of polyneuropathy."

Multiple sclerosis is an inflammatory disease where the myelin sheath covering the nerve cells in the central nervous system (brain and spinal cord) is damaged. Multiple sclerosis is a devastating illness that can manifest in many different ways including sudden blindness, weakness or paralysis in an extremity, as well as any abnormal neurological symptom.

Anything that disrupts the myelin sheath could conceivably be thought to cause or exacerbate multiple sclerosis. It is not beyond reason that statin use could cause multiple sclerosis when it is understood that cholesterol is a vital component of myelin. Amazingly, some have claimed that statins could treat MS via an anti-inflammatory mechanism.[29] However, other researchers have reported that statins do not prevent nor do they treat MS.[30] I will make a bold prediction here: Statins will never be shown to be an effective treatment for multiple sclerosis.

ALS AND STATINS

Amyotrophic lateral sclerosis (ALS) or Lou Gehrig's disease is a horrific neurodegenerative illness that affects the nerve cells in the brain and the spinal cord. ALS is characterized by a progressive degeneration of the motor neurons eventually leading to death. The incidence of ALS is two per 100,000 people. About 30,000 people in the U.S. suffer with ALS at any one time period. There is no known definitive cause of ALS. There were 334 cases of ALS reported to the FDA (FAERS) after those individuals took statin medications.

Abnormal lipid metabolism has been reported to cause ALS.[31] [32] Researchers compared the daily dietary intake, body weight, and serum lipid and glucose levels in ALS mice and wild-type controls at different stages of disease.[33] They found total cholesterol low-density lipoprotein (LDL) and LDL/high-density lipoprotein (HDL) ratio were significantly lower in ALS mice compared with controls. Further analysis found the low lipid levels were found in the presymptomatic stage of the disease. Furthermore, the low lipid levels were significantly greater in male but not female mice. The authors concluded, "Our findings suggest that hypolipidemia (low levels of cholesterol, LDL-cholesterol and other lipids) might be associated with the pathomechanism of ALS..."

Furthermore, other researchers have noticed an increase in ALS or ALS-like syndrome with statin therapy.[34] My THINCS colleagues, Mark R. Goldstein, M.D. and Luca Mascitelli, M.D., agree that statins may cause ALS or an ALS-like syndrome.[35] They describe an intricate mechanism where statins increase the immune system cells known as Tregs by inducing the transcription factor Forkhead box P3 (FoxP3). This effect may..."perpetuate neurodegenerative disorders by impairing neuroprotective autoimmunity.[36]

Drs. Goldstein and Mascitelli further describe how elevated glutamate levels in the brain have been associated with chronic neurodegenerative disorders including ALS as well as acute CNS trauma. Glutamate is an excitatory neurotransmitter which can stimulate the brain. However, it can also function as an excitotoxin which can cause nerve-cell inflammation and death. Excess glutamate levels have been associated with a host of neurodegenerative disorders including Alzheimer's disease and ALS. Glutamate is also found in foods as monosodium glutamate or MSG as a flavor enhancer. Unbelievably, MSG has also been placed into some vaccines. (Note: I would advise you to avoid all vaccines that contain MSG). Drs. Goldstein and Mascitelli state, "...we strongly agree...that statins should not be used in patients with ALS or ALS-like syndromes."

PARKINSON'S AND STATINS

Parkinson's disease is a devastating illness that generally affects 1% of people over the age of 50. Parkinson's disease can be caused by infections, exposure to environmental toxins such as pesticides, carbon monoxide, or the metal manganese.

The highest concentration of cholesterol occurs in the brain, where it is locally produced.[37] Cholesterol in the brain functions as an antioxidant and it helps to protect nerve cells from toxins. When toxin levels increase, both the brain and the body will increase their production of cholesterol. Therefore, any substance that interferes with the brain's or the body's ability to increase cholesterol production could be predicted to cause brain disorders such as Parkinson's disease.

Researchers prospectively studied plasma lipids and statin use in relation to Parkinson's disease in the Atherosclerosis Risk in Communities Study (ARIC).[38] Subjects had their statin use and lipid levels assessed at baseline and were followed for 11 years. The subjects who were using a statin before the study began were found to have a 139% (RR) increase in Parkinson's disease. Conversely, higher total cholesterol was associated with a lower risk for Parkinson's disease. Compared with the lowest tertile of average cholesterol, those in the highest tertile had a 57% lowered risk for developing Parkinson's disease. The authors concluded, "Statin use may be associated with a higher Parkinson's disease risk, whereas higher total cholesterol may be associated with a lower risk."

Similarly, another study found a lowered LDL-cholesterol level associated with a higher risk of Parkinson's disease.[39] Recall from Chapter 3 that the LDL-cholesterol level will parallel total cholesterol levels. Specifically, as compared to those with LDL-cholesterol levels above 138mg/dl, those with:

- LDL 115-137mg/dl had a 120% increased risk (RR) of Parkinson's disease

- LDL 93-114mg/dl had a 250% increased risk (RR) of Parkinson's disease

- LDL<92mg/dl had a 160% increased risk (RR) of Parkinson's disease

When you understand how important cholesterol is for the optimal functioning of the brain, it should be no surprise that statin drugs are associated with brain issues such as Parkinson's disease.

DIABETES AND STATINS

Diabetes is an independent risk factor for developing cardiovascular disease. Statins have been shown to increase the risk for type 2 (adult onset) diabetes by 10-12% with the risk directly related to the dose of the statin medication.[40] For over 20 years, it has been known that statins can adversely affect insulin secretion and sensitivity.[41] Surprisingly, the American College of Cardiology and the American Heart Association 2013 Cholesterol Guidelines recommend that all patients with diabetes who are 40-75 years of age should be placed on a moderate or high intensity statin medication to prevent or delay cardiovascular disease.[42]

You read that paragraph correctly. Statins increase the risk for diabetes. And, stronger statin medications increase the diabetes risk as compared to weaker ones. Diabetes is a risk for heart disease. Yet, The Powers-That-Be recommend high-dose statin therapy to diabetics to prevent heart disease. You are probably thinking (as am I) that we are, again, like Alice In Wonderland, where up is down and down is up.

The adverse drug reactions from statins in relationship to diabetes are as follows. Over a 10-year time period (2004-2014), the FAERS adverse drug reports of statins include:

- 14,463 cases of diabetes
- 27,367 cases of elevated blood sugar

ACUTE KIDNEY INJURY AND STATINS

Researchers studied over two million statin users over 40 years old and looked at each person hospitalized for acute kidney injury and matched them with ten controls.

The scientists found in patients with non-chronic kidney disease, current users of high potency statins were 34% more likely to be hospitalized with acute kidney injury within 120 days after starting treatment. Users of high potency statins with chronic kidney disease were found to have a 10% increase in admission rate. [43]

Statins are also well known to cause liver problems. From 2004-2014, there were 5548 cases of liver abnormalities reported to the FDA.

CANCER AND STATINS

Low cholesterol is a known risk factor for cancer. All the cholesterol-lowering medications from fibrates[44] to statins[45] [46]have been associated with an increased cancer rate. To be fair, there are other studies that have found no association between statins and cancer.

Animal studies have found cholesterol-lowering medications associated with cancer of the intestines, liver, thyroid, as well as lymphoma.[47] Researchers have concluded, "Most cholesterol-lowering medications cause or promote cancer in rodents. Patients to whom these drugs are prescribed...are exposed throughout many years to doses approaching those shown to be carcinogenic in animals."[48]

Some human statin studies have found an association between statin use and the development of cancer of the skin.[49] Other studies have found that the number of cancer deaths was three-fold higher in statin-treated patients who had a total cholesterol <160mg/dl when they were compared to those with higher cholesterol levels.[50]

Statins have been associated with an increase in cancer of the prostate[51], pancreas[52], and breast. The relationship between statin use and breast cancer will be covered in Chapter 10. Researchers have also pointed out that long-term use of statins may result in more aggressive cancers.[53]

Over a 10-year time period (2004-2014), the FAERS adverse drug reports of statins and cancer include:

- 1,515 cases of prostate cancer
- 2,608 cases of breast cancer

WHY AREN'T THE ADVERSE EFFECTS OF STATINS MORE COMMONLY KNOWN?

Recall that the statin drugs are the most profitable drugs in the history of the Big Pharma Cartel. Needless to say, Big Pharma has a financial interest to publish positive articles about statins. Nearly all of the published research on statins has focused on the benefits. Research scientists know a positive drug article will be more likely to be published as compared to a negative article.

The medical literature states that statin adverse effects are low. However, clinicians know the opposite is true; statin adverse effects are common. Research articles have acknowledged this disconnect.[54]

Part of this problem lies in how statin studies are performed. In *Therapeutics Initiatives*, it is explained that some statin studies recruit patients and put them in a "run-in period" when all patients are exposed to the drug prior to randomization and only those tolerating the drug are randomized.[55] Those initially suffering adverse effects are removed from the study.

Also, most health care workers discount statins as a cause of patient-reported side effects. One study looked at how physicians responded to their patients when presented with a possible adverse side effect of a statin medication. Out of 650 subjects, 87% spoke to their physician about the possible connection between statin use and their symptoms. The authors of this study stated, "Patients reported that they, and not the doctor, most commonly initiated the discussion regarding the possible connection of drug to symptom. Physicians were more likely to deny than affirm the possibility of a connection. Rejection of a possible connection was reported to occur even for symptoms with strong literature support for a drug connection, and even in patients for whom the symptom met presumptive literature-based criteria for probable or definite drug-adverse effect causality."[56] It is well known that the vast majority of adverse drug reactions are not reported to the FDA. In fact, the former head of the FDA estimated that less than 5% of all serious adverse drug reactions are reported to the FDA.[57]

FINAL THOUGHTS

The adverse drug reaction data on statins really speaks for itself. Once you understand the mechanism of the action of statin drugs and you comprehend how important cholesterol is to the body, these adverse event numbers should not be shocking. And, keep in mind that it is estimated that less than five percent of all adverse drug reactions are reported to the FDA.

What should be shocking is why so many health care providers as well as nearly every cardiologist prescribes these medications to the majority of patients they see.

Before taking a drug, it is important to educate yourself on how a drug works and what possible adverse effects are associated with the drug. You simply cannot rely on your health care provider to give you this information: most do not know how the drug actually works.

Remember, you are ultimately responsible for what drugs you take.

[1] JAMA. 2014.311(14):1416-23
[2] IBID. JAMA. 2014. 311.
[3] JAMA Int. Med. Published online Nov. 17, 2014. Accessed 12.7.14 from: http://archinte.jamanetwork.com/article.aspx?articleid=1935930
[4] http://fdable.com/
[5] JAMA. 1998:279.N. 15. 1200
[6] Accessed 1.28.15 from: http://www.rxlist.com/lipitor-drug/clinical-pharmacology.htm
[7] Accessed 1.28.15 from: https://www.crestortouchpoints.com/about-crestor/pharmacokinetics/
[8] BBA Molecular Basis of Disease, Vol. 1271, N. 1. May, 1995.
[9] Am J Cardiol. 2007;99:1409-1412
[10] Young, J. 5th Intl. CoQ10 FP-025.doc. Accessed 1.28.15 from: http://www.senpu.jp/coq10/pdf/jp-025.pdf
[11] *Journal of Clinical Pharmacology* **33** (3): 226–9. doi:10.1002/j.1552-4604.1993
[12] Atherosclerosis. 2007;195:e182-e189
[13] Am. J. of Clin. Nutr. 97:268-75. 2013
[14] *Circulation*. 2013;127:e6–e245
[15] IBID. Circulation. 2013:127
[16] *Circulation*. 2011;123(8):933–44
[17] Jpn. Heart J. 1976;17;32-42
[18] J Am Coll Cardiol 2008;52:1435–41
[19] Am. J. of Clin. Nutr. 97:268-275. 2013
[20] J. Am. Coll. Cardiol. 2000;35:816-7
[21] CMAJ. July 7, 2009. 181(1-2). E11-18
[22] Graveline, Duanne. The Statin Damage Crises. 2009
[23] Am. J. Med. May:108(7):538. 2000
[24] Gen Hosp. Psych. 2014. Sept-Oct;36(5):497-501
[25] Neurol. Res. 2014. Mar;36(3):247-54
[26] J. of Neurol. Sciences. 2014. Doi: 10.1016/jns.2014.11.013
[27] Nature Neuroscience. 8. 468-475. 2005
[28] Neurology. 2002:58:1333-37
[29] Weber, M. Statin in Multiple Sclerosis. Chapter 40 in Multiple Sclerosis Therapeutics. 4th Ed. 2011
[30] The Cochrane Library. Statins for Multiple Sclerosis. Dec 7, 2011
[31] Amyotrophic Lateral Sclerosis. 10: 113-17. 2009
[32] Neurology 70:1004-9. 2008
[33] PLoS ONE 6(3): e17985. doi:10.1371/journal.pone.0017985. 2011
[34] Drug Safety. 30(6): 515-525. 2007
[35] Drug Safety. 31(2): 181-82. 2008
[36] Drug Safety. IBID. 2008.
[37] Arteriosclerosis, Thrombosis, and Vascular Biology. 2004; 24: 806-815
[38] Movement Disorders. 2015. Published ahead of print. DOI: 10.1002/mds.25152

[39] Movement Disorders. 2007. Feb:22(3). p. 377
[40] J. Of Clin. Lipidology. 2014. 8. S17-s29
[41] Golstein, M., et al. Curr. Diab. Rep. 2013. DOI: 10,1007/s11892-013-0368-x
[42] Stone, NJ, et al. 2014. ACC/AHA Guidelines on the treatment of blood cholesterol to reduce atherosclerotic cardiovascular risk in adults. A report of the ACC/AHA task force on practice guidelines. Circulation. 129(25 Suppl. 2): s1-s45
[43] BMJ. 346:1880. 2013
[44] QJM. 103:202. 2010
[45] Lancet. 1994;344;1383-9
[46] Lancet. 2002;360.7-22
[47] JAMA. January 3, 1996. Vol. 275, n. 1
[48] JAMA. January 3, 1996. IBID
[49] Q.J.Med. doi:10.1093/qjmed/hcr243
[50] Circ. J. 66.1087-95. 2002
[51] Am. J. Epidem. 168:250-60. 2008
[52] Int. J. Med. Sci. 2015. Jan 22;12(3):223-33
[53] BJU Int. 2011;108. E211-6
[54] Cardiovasc. Drugs. 2008:8:373-418
[55] Therapeutics Initiative. Evidence Based Drug Therapy Statins. 89. April-May 2004.
[56] Drug Safety. 2007. 30(8): 669-75
[57] JAMA. Vol 269;21; June 2, 1993.

Chapter 10

Women and Statins

CHAPTER 10: INTRODUCTION

Women are often treated as second-class citizens when it comes to heart disease. Many women have their heart disease symptoms ignored by the medical profession as many health professionals are under the mistaken impression that heart disease only affects men. It can be difficult for a women who is suffering symptoms from heart disease to receive a proper diagnosis and treatment plan. To be fair, a woman's symptoms of heart disease are very different from a man's and can be more difficult to evaluate. My experience has shown that most women with heart disease do not present with the classical symptoms of chest pain, sweating, and difficult breathing that men do.

This chapter will review the use of statins in women and discuss their risks and benefits for women. All risks for statins are reported as relative risk unless other specified.

WOMEN: UNDERREPRESENTED IN HEART STUDIES

A woman tends to develop heart disease about ten years later in life than a man and a woman's risk of heart disease equals a man's risk at approximately age 70.

Many are under the impression that breast cancer kills more women than heart disease. That is not true. Heart disease is the leading cause of death of both men and women. In fact, in the U.S., 23.5% of all deaths of women in 2010 were due to heart disease. Cancer is next in line killing 22.1% of women. Approximately 350,000 women die from heart disease every year in the U.S.[1]

Since most health professionals are fixated on treating cholesterol levels, women are being treated with statin medications in ever-increasing numbers. It is estimated that nearly 25% of women and 30% of men over 45 years old presently take a statin medication. The new 2013 treatment guidelines for lowering cholesterol would markedly increase the numbers of both men and women who would qualify for lifelong statin therapy.

You would think, because so many women are taking—and many more qualify for taking—statin medications, that the research behind their use would clearly show a mortality and cardiovascular mortality benefit. Well, you would think wrong. Keep in mind who is funding these studies—Big Pharma. Big Pharma has every reason to recommend statins for both men and women; the more people that take them, the larger the profit will be for Big Pharma. The fact is, the studies on the benefits for statin therapy in women are abysmal. Keep in mind the statin research results in men are nothing to get excited about either.

The Search for Statin Indication in Women

Big Pharma has been on a quest to prove that statin use in women will be beneficial in preventing heart attacks and saving lives. Big Pharma would have you believe that statins are as effective for women as they are for men. They are not. What is true about statin use in women is that they:

- Do not prevent healthy women from having their first cardiac event
- Do not prevent death
- Increase the risk of diabetes
- May increase the risk of breast cancer

In fact, there is <u>not</u> a single published trial with a placebo group as a control that has found statins to significantly reduce mortality in women.[2]

PRIMARY PREVENTION USE OF STATINS IN WOMEN

Recall that primary prevention in statin therapy refers to using a statin to prevent a first cardiac event. The JUPITER trial studied the use of Crestor® in healthy men and women. The results for women in JUPITER were underwhelming as the 6,801 women included in the study were found to have no significant reduction in heart attacks, stroke and death when compared with the control group.[3]

A meta-analysis of eight trials which included 19,052 women and 30,194 men, looked at the gender benefits of statins in preventing cardiac outcomes in primary prevention. The authors reported that statins did not have a beneficial effect on mortality of both men and women in primary prevention over the 2.8 to 5.3 year study period. Furthermore, the scientists found statin therapy did not reduce the risk of coronary heart disease in women without a prior history of cardiovascular disease. They concluded, "Our study showed that statin therapy did not reduce the risk of total mortality in both men and women."[4]

Another meta-analysis of 6 trials, which included 11,435 women without cardiovascular disease, found that lipid-lowering therapy did not reduce total mortality, coronary heart disease mortality, non-fatal heart attacks, or coronary heart disease events.[5]

Scientists looked at the use of statins for primary prevention and the legal implications thereof. They found a lack of evidence for using statins in primary prevention in women. The authors state that the research on statins in women do not support "...approving or advertising statins as reducing heart attacks...for women." Furthermore, the authors questioned the use of direct-to-consumer marketing of statins without reporting that the "...inconclusive, and possibly contrary results in women."[6]

The same authors examined eight trials including 8,272 women with cardiovascular disease—this would be considered a secondary prevention analysis. Lipid lowering did not reduce total mortality in women with cardiovascular disease.[7]

The ASCOT study (reviewed in more detail in Chapter 7), found women treated with Lipitor® for 3.3 years had <u>more</u> cardiac events as compared to the control group.[8]

Women, Statins, and Diabetes

Statins have been shown to increase the risk of developing diabetes in women. The JUPITER study showed a significant 25% increase in the incidence of type 2 diabetes in women who were treated with a statin medication.[9]

The Women's Health Initiative (WHI) Study of 153,840 women found that statin use for three years was associated with a 71% increased risk of diabetes. This increased risk was observed for all types of statin medications. The authors concluded, "Statin medication use in postmenopausal women is associated with an increased risk for {diabetes}."[10]

Remember, in Chapter 7, I told you that absolute risk differences were much more important than relative risk differences in determining whether a therapy is beneficial—or in this case harmful—for a particular patient. Table 1 shows the data from the Women's Health Initiative (WHI) comparing the onset of diabetes in women who took a statin and those who did not.

Table 1: Data from WHI

Taking A Statin	% of New Onset Diabetes
Yes	9.93
No	6.41

The absolute risk difference between the two groups in Table 1 is 3.52% (9.93%-6.41%). The number needed to harm is:

$$1/.0352=28$$

That means that for every 28 women taking a statin medication, one will get diabetes (in this case, the number needed to harm). Now that may not sound like much, but health care providers should not be giving medications that cause serious problems like diabetes. It goes without saying that medications should be treating and preventing illnesses. Furthermore, diabetes increases the risk for heart disease—the exact thing they are trying to prevent by taking a statin!

STATINS AND CANCER

All classes of cholesterol-lowering medications have been associated with an increased risk of cancer. Low cholesterol levels are also associated with an increased risk of cancer. Furthermore, researchers have shown that diabetes is associated with cancer mortality.[11] Statins are known to increase insulin levels, which can enhance tumor cell proliferation through increasing the production of growth factors such as IGF-1.[12][13] I showed you earlier that statins increase the risk for diabetes, especially in women and the elderly.[14][15]

To be fair, the studies of statins and cancer risk have been inconsistent; not every study has shown an increased risk. In fact, some studies have shown a lowered risk [16][17][18] while others have shown an increased risk[19][20][21][22][23][24] and still others have shown no risk difference.

In 1996, an article in the Journal of the American Medical Association reported, "All members of the two most popular classes of lipid-lowering drugs (the fibrates and the statins) cause cancer in rodents, in some cases at levels of animal exposure close to those prescribed in humans. Evidence of carcinogenicity of lipid-lowering drugs from clinical trials in humans is inconclusive because of inconsistent results and insufficient duration of follow-up."[25]

The "inconsistent results" the researchers referred to might include the failure of researchers to monitor skin cancer incidence in statin studies. This is important because there is evidence that statin therapy causes an increased risk of non-melanoma skin cancer.[26] However, many of the recent statin studies have failed to include skin cancer (specifically squamous cell carcinoma) in their reports.[27] Furthermore, it takes many cancers ten or more years to develop. Most statin studies are not carried out that long.

Researchers designed a population-based case-control study of the two most common histologic subtypes of breast cancer: invasive ductal carcinoma (IDC) and invasive lobular carcinoma (ILC) among women 55-74 years of age living in the Seattle metropolitan area. They reported that current users of statins for ten years or longer had an 83% increased risk of IDC and a 97% increased risk of ILC compared with those who have never been users of statins.[28]

Thyroid cancer is increasing at epidemic rates, especially in women. When compared to controls, researchers reported a 40% increase risk of thyroid cancer in previous regular users of statin medications.[29]

WHY DOES BIG PHARMA HIDE THE DATA ON WOMEN?

Many studies on statins and women do not include the full data on gender-specific mortality. Many writers have complained about the ongoing problem of non-disclosure by Big Pharma.[30,31,32] One author pointed out many studies fail to report the mortality data in women including the Heart Protection Study (HPS), Prospective Study of Pravastatin in Elderly at Risk (PROSPER), and the Primary Prevention of Cardiovascular Disease with Pravastatin in Japan (MEGA) study.[33] Furthermore, in the studies that do provide full mortality statistics, the outcomes for women are poor; there is neither an absence of event nor mortality benefit for women.[34]

FINAL THOUGHTS

An article in The New York Times examined the issue of statin effectiveness in women.[35] In the article, a leading cardiologist stated, "We haven't shown that {statins} can prevent deaths, because we haven't enrolled enough women, and that's a crime. But, the absence of data isn't the same as negative data."

Wow. Read that statement again. A criticism that is constantly cast at those of us who practice holistic medicine is that there is a lack of data proving the effectiveness of the natural therapies which many of us espouse. (Those arguments are false—there is much data to the contrary).

Here, a leading cardiologist is stating that we have not enrolled enough women. How many women do they need? One million? A billion? The reason they need so many women is that an ineffective therapy requires a very large number of subjects in order to show a miniscule positive effect.

Yes, in the past, there were not enough women in cholesterol studies. That has changed in the past ten years. There are certainly enough women in the latest studies to draw a firm conclusion: statin drugs should be contraindicated for use in women. Statins drugs do not perform better than placebo at decreasing mortality—which should be the number one reason anyone takes a statin medication. When you throw in the adverse effects of statins, particularly the increased risk for diabetes, I say, "Fugetaboutit!".

[1] Accessed 1.15.14 from:
http://www.cdc.gov/nchs/data/nvsr/nvsr61/nvsr61_04.pdf
[2] Journal of Clinical Lipidology May-Jun;7(3): 222-24. (2013).
[3] NEJM. Nov. 20, 2008. Vol. 359 N. 21
[4] International Journal of Cardiology 138 (2010) 25–31
[5] JAMA. Vol. 291, n. 18. May 12, 2004
[6] J Empirical Legal Stud 2008;5:507–50
[7] IBID. JAMA. May 12, 2004
[8] Lancet. 2003;361:1149-1158.
[9] N. Eng. J. of Med. 2008;359:2195-07
[10] Arch. Int. Med. 2012:172(2):144-152
[11] Diabetes Care. 2012;35:1835-44
[12] Cancer Epidemiol Biomarkers Prev 2013;22:1923
[13] Integ. Cancer Ther. 2003. 2(4):315-29. 2003
[14] Curr. Diab. Rep. 12:381-90.2013
[15] Diabetes Care:36:a100-1. 2013
[16] Arch. Intern. Med. 160:2363-8. 2000
[17] J. of Women's Health. (Larchmt). 12:7:749-56. 2003
[18] J. Natl. Cancer Inst. 2006:98:700-7
[19] Arch. Int. Med. 153:1079-87. 1993
[20] J. Clin. Epidem. 56:280-5. 2003
[21] Int. J. Cancer. 114:643-7: 2005
[22] Br. J. Cancer. 2004:90:635-7
[23] J. Clin. Oncol. 2004:22:2388-94
[24] Cancer Epidemiol. Biomarkers Prev. 2007:16:4: 16-21
[25] JAMA. Vol. 275, N. 1. 1996
[26] Eur J Cancer 2008; 44: 2122-2132
[27] Transplant Immunology
Volume 23, Issue 4, August 2010, Pages 224–225
[28] Epidem. Biomarkers Prev. 22:1529-37. 2013
[29] Statin Use and Thyroid Cancer: A Population-Based Control Study. Doi: 10.1111/cen.12570. Clinical Endocrinology. 11.3.2014.
[30] Int J Cardiol 2010;138:25–31
[31] J Am Coll Cardiol 2004;44:1009–10
[32] JAMA 2004;291:2243–52
[33] In. J. of Card. Vol. 144, Issue 1. 9.24.2010
[34] Int. J. Cardiol. 2010;138:25-31
[35] NYT. May 5, 2014

Chapter 11

Cholesterol and Hormones

CHAPTER 11: INTRODUCTION

In Chapter 6, I discussed the biosynthetic pathway for cholesterol. Recall that there are multiple chemical reactions that occur in this pathway and that statins poison the enzyme HMG CoA Reductase, which is necessary to produce cholesterol. Therefore, statins are very effective at lowering cholesterol levels.

This chapter will review the adrenal and sex hormones. More information about bioidentical hormones can be found in my book, *The Miracle of Natural Hormones*.

Figure 1 illustrates the adrenal and sex hormone biosynthetic pathway. The adrenal glands are found adjacent to the kidneys and are necessary for producing many different hormones including: pregnenolone, DHEA, progesterone, estrogen, testosterone, and cortisol. The sex glands include the ovaries and the testicles. They produce estrogen and testosterone.

Note that the adrenal and sex hormone biochemical pathway begins from the fat-like substance cholesterol. Therefore, anything that lowers cholesterol levels is bound to affect this pathway. This chapter will discuss these hormones and how statin medications can adversely affect the body's ability to manufacture adrenal and sex hormones.

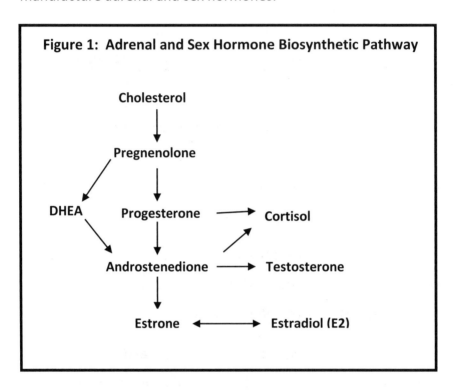

My father, Ellis, was the first patient I treated with bioidentical hormones. He had his first myocardial infarction (MI) or heart attack at age 42 and his first bypass surgery at age 50. Ellis' second bypass occurred at age 58. He had an angioplasty at age 60. Ellis never had his hormone levels checked during this entire time, yet he saw one of the best cardiologists in the area. My father suffered from frequent bouts of angina throughout this time period, and I never recall him looking or acting well as I was

growing up. Furthermore, his cholesterol levels were very high, always over 300 mg/dl and virtually unresponsive to cholesterol-lowering medications. When he was 63 years old, I checked his testosterone (no one had done so previously) and his thyroid hormone levels. His testosterone level and thyroid levels were extremely low. I placed him on Armour® thyroid hormone for a low thyroid state, and natural, bioidentical testosterone due to his low levels. From that moment on, he had virtually no symptoms of heart disease—a 25-year history of angina resolved within seven days and never returned. And, more importantly, he never felt or looked better. Furthermore, Ellis' cholesterol level, which had been elevated to over 300mg/dl on cholesterol-lowering medications, fell to less than 200mg/dl after starting the hormones. And, my father did not watch his diet nor did he ever exercise, much to my consternation. Shortly after starting this therapy, my parents took a trip with their high school friends Donna and Leonard. Donna phoned me after the trip. She asked me what I was prescribing for my father. When I asked her why, she replied, "David, I haven't seen your father look this good in 30 years; I want to give Leonard the same thing." I believe my father may have been able to avoid much of his heart disease history if he had been placed on natural, bioidentical hormones earlier in his life.

One final note on my father. Shortly after treating him

with thyroid hormone and testosterone, I checked his other adrenal hormones including DHEA, pregnenolone, and progesterone. His levels were virtually undetectable in all the laboratory tests. When I placed him on small amounts of DHEA (10mg/day), pregnenolone (25mg/day) and progesterone (10mg/day) his health further improved. My father took all of these bioidentical hormones until he died at age 70. My father was also treated with vitamins and minerals for nutritional deficiencies. I have no doubt that bioidentical hormone supplementation markedly improved his lifestyle and extended his lifespan.

My father's case history is perfect for illustrating why elevated cholesterol levels should not be treated with medications—like statins–that poison the cholesterol biosynthetic pathway. My father did not suffer from statin-deficiency syndrome; he was suffering from hormonal and nutritional imbalances.

Nearly all doctors today believe that an elevated cholesterol level causes heart disease. However, I do not believe that statement. The human body is a marvelous invention. It is not designed to self-destruct. My clinical experience has clearly shown that, in most cases of hypercholesterolemia, the body is appropriately producing elevated cholesterol because of what is happening in the body. Keep in mind that cholesterol is a vital, essential substance produced in the body.

HEAVY METALS AND CHOLESTEROL

Cholesterol has anti-inflammatory properties. In cases of excess inflammation from infections or injury, the body's natural response is to produce more cholesterol to protect the cell membranes and neurological tissues. Anything that produces inflammation can cause the body to produce excess amounts of cholesterol in order to protect the vital organs, including the brain, from the inflammatory toxins. In these examples, the worst thing a doctor could do is to prescribe a drug which poisons the cholesterol biosynthetic pathway.

Heavy metal toxicity—occurring from mercury, lead, arsenic, cadmium, or nickel exposure–can cause the body to produce too much cholesterol. Cholesterol helps protect the cell membrane and the cell machinery from the toxic effects of heavy metals. In fact, the sickest patients suffering with a heavy metal toxicity are the ones who cannot increase their cholesterol production. I do not institute a detoxification program for patients with low cholesterol (below 150mg/dl) who have a heavy metal toxicity. In this situation, the first step is to increase cholesterol levels. This can be accomplished through improving the diet by increasing the intake of healthy sources of protein and fat, as well as undergoing liver detoxification. A detoxification program can be started after cholesterol levels rise above 150mg/dl. My clinical experience has clearly shown that elevated cholesterol levels will naturally reduce when a heavy metal toxic patient is appropriately detoxified. I, along with my partners, have formulated a liver detoxification formula known as Total Liver Care (TLC). The Appendix will provide more information about TLC.

It is very important for health care professionals to search for the underlying cause of an elevated cholesterol level. If the body has a statin-deficiency syndrome, then perhaps a statin is warranted. In all my years of practicing medicine, I have yet to see a statin-deficiency syndrome patient. If a cholesterol level is elevated, a thorough workup should be initiated to determine why the body is having to produce excess amounts of cholesterol.

ELEVATED CHOLESTEROL AND HORMONES

I have found that many patients produce excess amounts of cholesterol when they are deficient in the sex and adrenal hormones. Recall from Figure 1 that all the sex and adrenal hormones are produced downstream from cholesterol.

My theory is that adrenal and sex hormone-deficient

patients have elevated cholesterol due to the body appropriately trying to add more substrate—in this case cholesterol—to the pathway in order to stimulate the increased production of adrenal and sex hormones.

Recall my father's story. His cholesterol was always elevated over 300mg/dl. He also had insufficient production of the adrenal and sex hormones. When he corrected the hormonal deficit with bioidentical, natural hormones, his cholesterol level fell below 200mg/dl—without changing his diet or exercising. The drop in total cholesterol in my father's case can only be attributed to one thing: the use of bioidentical hormones which corrected a hormonal imbalance. The bioidentical hormones—testosterone and thyroid hormone—corrected the hypoadrenal and hypothyroid state he was suffering from which, in turn, allowed his body to reduce its excess production of cholesterol. I know that thyroid hormone is not in this pathway, but a well-regulated thyroid is vitally important for optimizing cholesterol levels and adrenal hormone function. More about thyroid function and cholesterol levels can be found in Chapter 12 and in my book, *Overcoming Thyroid Disorders*.

Since treating my father, I have successfully treated thousands of patients with bioidentical hormones. It is a routine finding in my practice (as well as that of my partners Drs. Ng and Nusbaum) that elevated cholesterol levels fall when the adrenal and sex hormones–as well as the thyroid– are balanced.

Testosterone

There are numerous studies linking atherosclerosis and coronary artery disease to low testosterone levels. A study by researchers from Columbia University's College of Physicians and Surgeons found those with low concentrations of testosterone in the blood were more likely to have atherosclerosis documented by angiography.[1] Moller, a Danish physician, found that 83% of patients' cholesterol levels fell significantly while taking testosterone. On average, the cholesterol level after testosterone therapy was 74% of the pretreatment condition.[2] I'm sure these patients felt a lot better on this therapy compared to conventional medicine's approach of cholesterol-lowering medications and their side effects which include nausea, abdominal pain, gall bladder disease, a decreased libido, liver problems, neurological disorders, muscle aches and pains, as well as dementia.

Several studies document low testosterone levels associated with high triglycerides and LDL cholesterol. Other studies have shown that normal testosterone levels are associated with increased HDL cholesterol, which is thought to protect against atherosclerosis. Testosterone has been shown to enhance HDL-cholesterol induced reverse cholesterol transport which helps remove cholesterol from the circulation and return it to the liver.[3]

In my practice, through the use of bioidentical, natural hormones like natural testosterone, I have witnessed the same type of results that my father experienced: a lowering of cholesterol levels and an improvement in the symptoms of coronary artery disease. These results have been repeated over and over in my practice. I believe that anyone who suffers from coronary artery disease should have a testosterone level checked just as quickly as a physician would investigate a cholesterol level. In fact, testosterone and other hormones should be investigated before starting a workup on cholesterol. When low testosterone levels are adequately treated, many times, coronary artery disease will improve.

Researchers have estimated that over a 20-year period, testosterone deficiency is associated with:[4]

- 1.3 million new cases of cardiovascular disease
- 1.1 million cases of diabetes
- Over 600,000 osteoporosis-related fractures

It is not just an increased risk of heart disease that is associated with low testosterone levels. Symptoms of low testosterone include depression, erectile dysfunction, fatigue, loss of libido, as well as muscle aches and pains. Testosterone deficiency is also associated with an increased risk of metabolic syndrome and diabetes. Not surprisingly, statin medication's adverse effects mimic low testosterone symptoms. Furthermore, low testosterone levels and statin use are both associated with an increased risk for diabetes.

Once you understand the adrenal and sex hormone biochemical pathway (Figure 1, page 208), you could predict that statin use will lower testosterone and other important hormone levels. That is exactly what happens.

Researchers studied 3,484 men with erectile dysfunction.[5] [6] As compared to men not treated with statins, those treated with statins—primarily Zocor® or Lipitor®—were found to have significantly lowered testosterone levels. In fact, the men treated with statins were twice as likely to have low testosterone. Another study found statin use associated with significantly lowered testosterone levels as compared to subjects not taking a statin medication.[7]

Nearly 20,000 hypogonadal (low testosterone-producing) men received testosterone over a five-year period. Researchers reported that the risk of heart attack was seven-fold lower and the risk of stroke was nine-fold lower when the testosterone treated men were compared with samples from the general population.[8]

Another study compared 6,355 men treated with testosterone injections with matched controls. Testosterone therapy was associated with a 16% reduced risk of heart attack. Men in the highest quartile of risk had a 31% reduced risk of heart attack. The authors summarized the study by stating, "For men with a high myocardial infarction {heart attack} risk, testosterone use was modestly protective against myocardial infarction."[9]

Testosterone Treatment

Once a work-up has confirmed a low testosterone level, testosterone therapy should be considered. I suggest using bioidentical, natural testosterone either in injectable or topical versions. I strongly caution against using oral testosterone as this method has been associated with adverse effects such as an increased risk for cancer. The adverse effects for oral dosing do not occur with either topical or injectable forms of testosterone because these methods avoid the first-pass effect of the liver.

As I have indicated, I only use natural testosterone because it more closely mimics the body's own production of testosterone versus the synthetic derivatives of testosterone. Doses for women usually average 0.5-2 mg per day. For men, doses usually range from 40-120 mg per day. I prefer to use testosterone in cream form, as it is well absorbed through the skin. However, injectable sources of testosterone can also be used. I recommend using USP grade micronized natural testosterone made by a compounding pharmacist. Adverse effects of testosterone include acne, hair loss, and moodiness. These side effects are much more common in women than in men. Adjusting the dosage of testosterone usually takes care of these adverse effects.

Any testosterone therapy should be closely followed with blood tests on a regular basis. These tests should include a hemoglobin analysis, free and total testosterone levels as well as estradiol and total estrogen levels.

DHEA

DHEA is an acronym for dehydroepiandrosterone. It is an androgen hormone produced in the adrenal glands. DHEA is secreted into the bloodstream where it is converted in the liver to DHEA-sulfate (DHEA-S). All DHEA levels mentioned in this book are in the sulfated form of DHEA—DHEA-S. For clinical purposes, I have found laboratory testing for DHEA-S to be the most accurate measure of DHEA.

DHEA, being an androgen hormone, helps stimulate muscle tissue and keeps muscles strong. Furthermore, optimal DHEA levels are needed for maintaining libido, energy, and brain function. I have found DHEA therapy extremely helpful for those suffering with headaches, including migraine headaches, allergies and asthma, as well as autoimmune illnesses. DHEA can also be useful for treating conditions associated with fatigue as well as muscle aches and pains.

I have seen a direct correlation between low DHEA levels and fibromyalgia. Fibromyalgia is associated with muscle aches and pains along with fatigue. There are many conditions associated with low DHEA levels including autoimmune illnesses, cancer, and many other degenerative conditions. Since DHEA stimulates muscle growth and repair, it can be useful for any condition that affects the muscles of the body.

DHEA levels peak at approximately 20-25 years of age and gradually decline as we get older. Furthermore, chronic illness can hasten the age-related decline of DHEA.

DHEA AND STATINS

Stains are well-known for their adverse side effects to the muscles of the body. In Chapter 6, I discussed how statins interfere with CoQ10 production and how CoQ10 is needed for proper muscle function. Statin myopathy is the medical term for statin-induced muscle aches and pains.

I have found small amounts of DHEA can help a patient overcome statin myopathy if they do not continue to take the statin medication. However, DHEA therapy does not help every case of statin myopathy. The best results with DHEA occur when it is taken along with the adrenal hormone pregnenolone, which will be discussed next. Average doses of DHEA for most women range from 5-10mg/day and for men, the average is 10-20mg/day. There are very few minor adverse effects with DHEA. The most common adverse effect is moodiness and acne. It occurs in much less than 1% of the people who take it. Adverse effects with DHEA are easily treated by adjusting the dosage.

PREGNENOLONE

As can be seen from Figure 1, pregnenolone is the precursor hormone for the adrenal hormones. In fact, it is often referred to as the mother hormone as all adrenal and sex hormones are produced downstream from pregnenolone. Pregnenolone is produced in both the brain and adrenal glands. In fact, pregnenolone levels in the brain are much higher than they are in the peripheral tissues.[10] Pregnenolone has been shown to affect many of the neurotransmitters in the brain. Pregnenolone levels, like the other hormones mentioned in this book, decline with age. At age 75, there is a 65% reduction in pregnenolone production in the body as compared to levels at age 35.[11] I have found pregnenolone particularly useful in treating memory problems, fatigue, and depression.

As mentioned in Chapter 9, statin drugs are associated with brain dysfunction. This could easily be predicted by looking at the biochemical pathways and how statins disrupt these pathways. As can be seen from Figure 1, statin use can be predicted to lower pregnenolone levels as it will lower cholesterol levels. Lowered pregnenolone levels would be predicted to affect the muscles and the brain. Pregnenolone, similarly to DHEA and testosterone, is an androgen hormone which helps maintain and optimize muscle function.

Pregnenolone has a positive, synergistic effect when it is used with DHEA. I rarely use pregnenolone without the concurrent use of DHEA. Average doses of pregnenolone in women range from 10-25mg/day and in men, from 25-75mg/day. There are very few side effects from taking pregnenolone. The most common adverse effect is moodiness that is easily treated by adjusting the dosage.

PROGESTERONE

In women, progesterone is produced in both the ovaries and the adrenal glands. Large amounts of progesterone are produced in the luteal phase of the menstrual cycle. Men produce tiny amounts of progesterone from the testicles as well as the adrenal glands.

Progesterone is a natural diuretic and a natural antidepressant. It also helps convert inactive to active thyroid hormone. Progesterone is also very helpful for treating PMS and menopausal symptoms. Progesterone has anticancer properties and can normalize and help maintain appropriate blood sugar levels.

As can be seen from Figure 1, progesterone is produced downstream from cholesterol. Therefore, anything that impedes cholesterol production could be expected to negatively impact progesterone production.

Statin drugs, since they disrupt the production of cholesterol, should be expected to decrease the production of progesterone. And they do. All cholesterol drugs—older (fibrates) and newer (statins)—have been associated with increased cancer rates. Breast cancer was shown to increase by 1,200% in statin users.[12] To be fair, there are studies that show both a positive and negative association of statins and cancer. However, there are studies which show a five-fold increased risk in breast cancer in women deficient in progesterone. Furthermore, the same study found a ten-fold increased risk in developing cancer of any sort in women deficient in progesterone.[13] If a lowered progesterone level is truly associated with an increased risk of cancer, it should be no surprise that statin medications would be associated with an increased risk of cancer since statins will lower progesterone levels.

Both women and men require adequate progesterone levels. Progesterone is best used in a topical form as it is easily absorbed through the skin. Average doses of progesterone for women range from 10-100mg/day and for men from 5-10mg/day. When using progesterone, it is important to use bioidentical, natural versions of progesterone. The more commonly prescribed synthetic forms of progesterone found in birth control pills and many conventional hormonal preparations are associated with serious adverse effects including an increased risk of breast cancer, blood clots, heart disease, and Alzheimer's. All forms of synthetic progesterone should be avoided.

ESTROGENS

Estrogens are produced in both the adrenal glands and the sex glands in men and women. As compared to men, women produce larger quantities of estrogen. Estrogen can help women with menopausal symptoms including hot flashes and moodiness. In women, bioidentical, natural estrogens can help keep skin smooth and improve brain function.

Similarly to the other hormones discussed, estrogen production can be expected to decline with statin use. Statin use is associated with brain dysfunction including loss of memory, depression, anxiety, and moodiness. All of these symptoms can be associated with estrogen deficiency in women.

When using estrogen therapy, I suggest using bioidentical, natural versions of estrogen as they are much safer than synthetic forms such as Premarin®. Estrogen should never be taken orally as studies have clearly shown severe adverse effects with oral dosing. Oral dosing of estrogen causes it to be exposed to a first-pass effect in the liver which produces toxic estrogen byproducts. These toxic estrogen metabolites have been associated with an increased cancer risk. Topical versions of estrogen do not have this toxicity.

I have been successfully using topical versions of bioidentical, natural estrogen for over 20 years. Doses for women can range from 0.5-2.0mg/day. I suggest using estrogen from a compounding pharmacist who is skilled with dispensing bioidentical, natural estrogen.

One final note on estrogen therapy. Estrogen therapy should generally be used with progesterone. Conventional doctors are under the mistaken notion that women without a uterus do not need progesterone. They are wrong. Estrogen therapy works best when combined with natural, bioidentical progesterone.

FINAL THOUGHTS

After treating my father with bioidentical, natural testosterone and thyroid hormone I changed my practice. How could I not change it? My father's improved health was the impetus I needed to begin my quest to study natural therapies.

Since treating my father, I have treated thousands of patients with natural items. From what I have seen I can state, with authority, that physicians need to go back to their biochemical books and study the pathways. We need to support these pathways, not poison them.

Statins disrupt the adrenal and sex hormone pathways. Studying the effects of an imbalanced hormonal system should lead any health care practitioner to refuse to prescribe a statin drug.

The conclusions of studies may mislead. Statistics may lie. But biochemistry does not lie. We should be supporting the basic functions of the body. The use of bioidentical, natural hormones along with other natural therapies that help restore hormonal balance can provide miraculous results. I see them occur regularly in my practice.

[1] Fackelmann, K.A. Science News, May 28, 1994;145:340

[2] Moller, Jens *Cholesterol, Interactions with Testosterone and Cortisol in Cardiovascular Diseases.* Springer-Verlag, 1987.

[3] Annu. Rev. Med. 2003;54:321-41

[4] J. Sex. Med. 2013;10:562-69

[5] J. of Sex. Med. Vol. 7, Issue 4, part 1. p. 1547-56. April, 2010

[6] Accessed 1.2.14 from: http://www.webmd.com/erectile-dysfunction/news/20100416/statins_may_lower_testosterone_libido

[7] Urology. 76(5): 2010. p. 1048

[8] Presented at AACE 23rd Annual Scientific and Clinical Congress. May 2014. Accessed from: www.medscape.com/viewarticle/825326. January 1, 2015

[9] Annals of Pharm. 2014. Doi: 10.117710600028014539918

[10] Sahelian, Ray. *Pregnenolone, Nature's Feel Good Hormone.* Avery Publishing. 1997

[11] Roberts, Eugene. Pregnenolone-From Selye to Alzheimer and a Model of the pregnenolone sulfate binding site on the GABA Receptor. Biochemical Pharmacology, Vol. 49, No. 1. P. 1-16, 1995

[12] N.Eng. J. of Med. 385:1001-9. 1996

[13] Am.J. Epid. 114:1981. p. 209-217

Chapter 12

Cholesterol and Hypothyroidism

CHAPTER 12: INTRODUCTION

For over 70 years, it has been known that cholesterol levels are intricately related to thyroid function. For over 100 years, a low thyroid condition—hypothyroidism—has been linked to an increased risk of heart disease. It is sad that most, if not all, cardiologists fail to investigate the functioning of the thyroid gland when a new cardiac patient shows up at their office. Unfortunately, they are too busy prescribing statin medications at the first visit—regardless of what a patient's cholesterol level is. As I stated before, that would be appropriate if the patient was suffering from a statin-deficiency syndrome, but I have yet to see a patient with that.

This chapter will review the thyroid gland and its relationship to both cholesterol levels and the development of heart disease.

PHYSIOLOGY OF THE THYROID GLAND

The thyroid gland sits in the lower part of the neck and weighs about 1.5 ounces. It produces approximately one teaspoon of thyroid hormone per year. That teaspoon of thyroid hormone is necessary to drive the metabolic rate of every cell in the body. Every cell has thyroid receptors and requires optimal thyroid hormone levels to function optimally. It is impossible for the body to function optimally when there is inadequate thyroid hormone present.

Hypothyroidism is the term used for an inadequate supply of thyroid hormone in the body. When hypothyroidism is present, a constellation of symptoms develop. Table 1 lists the signs and symptoms of hypothyroidism.

HOW COMMON IS HYPOTHYROIDISM?

In the United States, the prevalence of hypothyroidism is staggering. The Colorado Thyroid Disease Prevalence Study estimated that the rate of hypothyroidism in the general population was approximately 10%.[1] In the United States, this correlates to 16 million adults who may have an undiagnosed hypothyroid condition. Although this study used blood testing alone to diagnose a hypothyroid condition, my research has clearly shown that relying solely on blood tests for this diagnosis will result in missing approximately 30% of those who have a hypothyroid condition. A holistic approach, which takes into account the laboratory tests, and the basal body temperatures, as well as the patient's signs and symptoms will identify many more individuals suffering from hypothyroidism.

Table 1: Signs and Symptoms of Hypothyroidism

Brain fog	Hoarseness
Brittle nails	Hypotension
Cold hands and feet	Inability to concentrate
Cold intolerance	Infertility
Constipation	Menstrual irregularities
Depression	
Difficulty swallowing	Muscle cramps
Dry skin	Muscle weakness
Elevated cholesterol	Nervousness
Essential hypertension	Poor memory
Eyelid swelling	Puffy eyes
Fatigue	Slower heartbeat
Hair loss	Throat pain

More information about this approach can be found in my book, *Overcoming Thyroid Disorders*. It is my opinion that the true figure for hypothyroidism is closer to 40% of the population or approximately 128 million adult Americans. Since hypothyroidism can cause elevated cholesterol levels and heart disease, I feel that many patients with heart disease are being misdiagnosed as statin-deficiency patients. As I previously stated, cardiac patients would be better served to have a complete hormonal and nutritional workup rather than just routinely starting them on cholesterol-lowering medications.

PHYSIOLOGY OF THE THYROID GLAND

To understand the importance of thyroid functioning and its relationship to heart disease and cholesterol, you have to understand the physiology behind the thyroid gland.

The thyroid gland produces two major hormones, Thyroxine (T4) and Triiodothyronine (T3) (see Figure 1, Page 233). These two hormones work inside the cells of the body, primarily influencing the metabolism of the cells. In other words, thyroid hormone helps the cell machinery produce energy. When there is an adequate amount of thyroid hormone, the cell machinery functions normally and the metabolism of the cells (and the body) occurs at a normal level. When there is an inadequate amount of

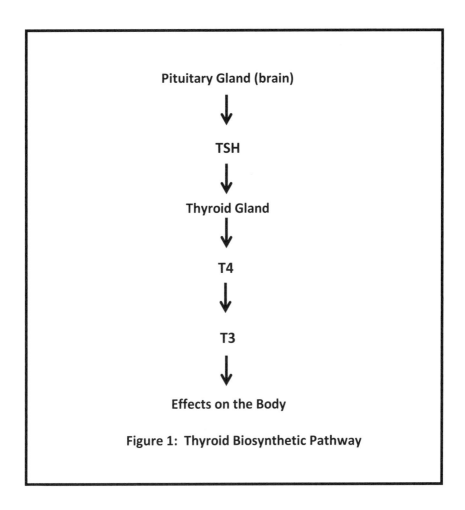

Figure 1: Thyroid Biosynthetic Pathway

thyroid hormone produced (i.e., hypothyroidism), the metabolism of the cells (and the body) will decline, and the signs and symptoms of hypothyroidism will be present.

The thyroid produces much more T4 (approximately 80%) than T3 (approximately 20%). T3 is much more active than T4 (about 300% more active)[2] and T3 is the thyroid hormone that actually increases the metabolism inside the cells. The majority of T4 is actually converted into T3 inside the cells of the body.

HOW IS THE THYROID GLAND STIMULATED?

A pituitary hormone, known as thyroid stimulating hormone or TSH (See Figure 1) stimulates the thyroid gland. When TSH is secreted from the pituitary gland, it causes the thyroid gland to release thyroid hormone. TSH is very sensitive to both T4 and to T3. When the body has adequate amounts of thyroid hormone available, TSH levels are lowered so that the thyroid gland can lower its production of hormones.

HOW IS HYPOTHYROIDISM DIAGNOSED? THE CONVENTIONAL APPROACH

This section is divided into the **conventional** diagnosis and the **holistic** diagnosis of hypothyroidism. The **conventional** approach to diagnosing hypothyroidism primarily revolves around the measurement of a single thyroid blood test–the thyroid stimulating hormone (TSH) test.

If the TSH is elevated, it is a sign that the pituitary gland is sensing a low thyroid hormone level in the body, and the TSH is being secreted in order to stimulate the thyroid gland to produce more thyroid hormone. If the TSH test is normal, many physicians believe that automatically rules out a hypothyroid state. See Figure 2 for TSH reference ranges.

Figure 2: TSH Ranges

TSH Reference Range: 0.4-4.5mIU/L
TSH Hypothyroid Range: >4.5mIU/L

The Problems with the TSH Test

The TSH test has been the "gold standard" in conventional medicine for diagnosing hypothyroidism for over 30 years. The reference range for the TSH test reported in most laboratories is from 0.4-4.5mIU/L. When TSH values fall above this range (i.e., >4.5mIU/L), a diagnosis of hypothyroidism is given. This reference range was established to include 95% of the population. Therefore, 5% of the population, which falls outside of this reference range, would be classified as having a thyroid disorder.

However, as reported in the Colorado Thyroid Study (mentioned above), many researchers believe that the true incidence of hypothyroidism is significantly higher than 5%. Dr. A.P. Weetman, professor of medicine, wrote in the British Medical Journal, "Even within the reference range of around 0.5-4.5mIU/L, a high thyroid stimulating hormone concentration (>2mIU/L) was associated with an increased risk of future hypothyroidism. The simplest explanation is that thyroid disease is so common that many people predisposed to thyroid failure are included in a laboratory's reference population. This raises the question whether thyroid replacement is appropriate in patients with thyroid stimulating hormone levels above 2mIU/L. The high frequency of overt and subclinical hypothyroidism observed raises another contentious issue--namely, whether screening for hypothyroidism is worthwhile."[3]

Therese Hertoghe, a Belgian endocrinologist, also feels that the TSH test is not sensitive enough in identifying a hypothyroid condition. In Dr. Hertoghe's experience, the TSH test may only identify 2-5% of hypothyroid individuals.[4] Dr. Hertoghe recommends correlating the blood test results with the clinical picture in order to secure an accurate diagnosis of hypothyroidism.

After over 20 years of practicing medicine, it has become clear to me that relying solely on the TSH test will result in under-diagnosing many individuals who are suffering from hypothyroidism—up to 30% of the population.

The TSH reference range (See Figure 2) is much too large. After diagnosing and treating thousands of patients for thyroid conditions, I have found that the optimal TSH reference range is from 0.5-2.0mIU/L. A TSH above 2.0mIU/L may indicate a hypothyroid condition.

THE RELATIONSHIP OF HYPOTHYROIDISM TO HEART DISEASE

Hypothyroidism was first described in the Western world in the nineteenth century. It wasn't until 1891 that the effective treatment of hypothyroidism with subcutaneous injections of thyroid extract was reported by Dr. George Murray in England. Myxedema refers to a severely low-thyroid state. This was described throughout the medical literature in the nineteenth and early twentieth Centuries. Atherosclerosis and heart attacks are a common finding of myxedematous and hypothyroid patients.

Hypothyroidism, The Unsuspected Illness is a book that was written in 1976 by Dr. Broda Barnes. Dr. Barnes wrote about his frustration with the commonly used thyroid function tests—which included the TSH test. Dr. Barnes felt that relying on the TSH test to diagnose a hypothyroid condition will cause many physicians to miss the diagnosis. He felt the TSH was an insensitive marker for hypothyroidism.

When Dr. Barnes wrote his book in 1976, he felt that most cardiologists were missing the underlying cause of heart disease. At that time, as it is now, heart disease was killing people at epidemic rates. Dr. Barnes felt that the cardiologists were erroneously focused on cholesterol and fat in the diet as the culprits. He spent many years researching the cause of heart disease.

Dr. Barnes' research took him to Graz, Austria. Dr. Barnes reviewed over 70,000 autopsy records in order to compare the cause of deaths that occurred between 1930 and 1970 in Graz, Austria. Dr. Barnes found that in 1930, before the advent of antibiotics, most deaths were due to infections and these deaths occurred at a relatively young age, less than 50 years old. Deaths from heart attacks were rare. In 1930, infection was effectively killing off the weak at a young age.

By 1970, due to the use of antibiotics, infections were causing fewer deaths than in 1930. However, deaths from heart attacks had increased 1,000 percent since 1930. Compared to 1930, in 1970 people were surviving to an older age and dying of a new cause—heart attacks. Dr. Barnes' hypothesis was that, "Either something new had entered the picture to cause the increase [in heart attacks], or those surviving premature death from infections were prone to develop heart disease. Careful study of the autopsy protocols indicated that the latter was true."[5]

The connection between the young individuals who died of infections in 1930 and the older individuals who died of heart attacks in 1970 was found in Dr. Barnes' research. The autopsy reports reviewed by Dr. Barnes showed that both groups, the young who died in 1930 and the old who died in 1970, had signs of advanced coronary artery disease. The only connection Dr. Barnes could draw to explain the cause of death in both groups was that both groups were suffering from the same problem: hypothyroidism.

After the advent of antibiotics, the hypothyroid population now began surviving infections and living to an older age. They began procreating, therefore creating new generations of hypothyroid individuals. As this group of people lived to an older age, now surviving infections through the use of antibiotics, the ravages of hypothyroidism began affecting them. This often took the form of coronary artery disease.

It is well known that the immune system does not function optimally in a hypothyroid individual, therefore increasing the risk of infection. The use of antibiotics often enables the hypothyroid individual to overcome an acute illness, as illustrated in Dr. Barnes' study. However, long-standing hypothyroidism, untreated over many years, will predispose the individual to develop coronary artery disease as well as other signs of hypothyroidism.

HIGH CHOLESTEROL AND HEART DISEASE

Coronary artery disease is the number one killer in this country. It has been the number one killer since antibiotics were introduced after World War II. Tens of millions of dollars have been spent studying why coronary artery disease affects such a wide range of the population. High cholesterol levels have been implicated as the cause of death due to heart disease. When a patient sees their doctor today, it is customary to have their cholesterol level checked. If the cholesterol level is high, the physician is quick to prescribe a cholesterol-lowering drug. But, perhaps the elevated cholesterol is only the symptom of another problem: hypothyroidism.

It has been known for over 70 years that hypothyroidism predisposes one to have high cholesterol levels. As I stated before, if a diagnosis of high cholesterol is made, then a proper search for an underlying cause of the high cholesterol should be conducted.

I have treated thousands of individuals with high cholesterol levels diagnosed by other physicians. Again, If there is an elevated cholesterol level present, then a thorough investigation should be undertaken to discover why there is a hypercholesterolemic situation. My clinical experience has clearly shown that many of these hypercholesterolemic patients are not suffering from a statin-deficiency situation. I have found that a large percentage of individuals with elevated cholesterol levels have thyroid and other hormonal imbalances present. Correcting the hormonal imbalance(s) in these patients oftentimes will correct the hypercholesterolemic problem without the use of a drug therapy.

At this point, it is important to note that statins do not treat hypothyroidism.

It is too bad that nearly all cardiologists are fixated on their patients' cholesterol levels. Yes, cardiac patients can have high cholesterol levels. However, high cholesterol is not a diagnosis of anything. It is a symptom of something wrong in the body. In many cases it is the "idiot light" of hypothyroidism.

HOW IS HYPOTHYROIDISM TREATED?

Once a diagnosis of hypothyroidism is made, the next step is to figure out what is causing the hypothyroid condition. This can be complex as there are many factors that can cause the thyroid to become underactive. These are listed in Table 2.

Each of the items listed in Table 2 can cause hypothyroidism. It is beyond the scope of this book to cover each of these items. More information on each of these causes can be found in *Overcoming Thyroid Disorders.*

The most common cause of hypothyroidism, by far, is iodine deficiency. In any case of hypothyroidism or heart disease, it is important to evaluate the iodine status of the individual. Low iodine is, unfortunately, the norm. I (along with my partners) have tested over 6,000 patients and we have found iodine

Table 2: Factors Associated with Hypothyroidism

Advanced age

Alpha-Lipoic Acid

Anti-TPO antibodies

Chronic illness

Cigarette smoking

Drugs (propylthiouracil, methimazole, dexamethasone, propranolol, amiodarone, birth control pills, estrogens, lithium)

External radiation

Fasting

Growth hormone deficiency

Heavy metal toxicity including mercury toxicity

Hemochromatosis

High stress

Iodinated cholestographic agents (used in x-ray procedures)

Iodine deficiency

Low adrenal states

Malnutrition

Mineral and vitamin deficiencies (iodine, selenium, vitamins A, B6 and B12)

Non-fermented soy ingestion

Physical trauma

Postoperative state

deficiency is occurring in over 96% of them. Iodine deficiency will be covered in the next chapter.

IF YOU THINK YOU HAVE A THYROID CONDITION, WHAT CAN YOU DO?

Unfortunately, most conventional doctors do not understand the connection between cholesterol levels and the thyroid gland. If you are told that you have high cholesterol and should take a statin medication, you should ask your doctor to check your thyroid function. If you are seeing a conventional doctor, chances are they do not know how to properly evaluate your thyroid status. It is best to work with a doctor knowledgeable about natural, bioidentical hormones and the way hormonal imbalances relate to cholesterol production. In the Appendix I will provide you with a resource to find a holistic practitioner. It may take you some time to find the right one, but it is worth it.

Final Thoughts

A high cholesterol level should be considered a warning light telling you that something is wrong. The doctors from the previous generation understood this connection. Unfortunately, most physicians today do not.

Cholesterol could be elevated for a number of reasons including a poor diet, having too much inflammation, and hypothyroidism. A high cholesterol level should cause your health care provider to begin a search for the reason why it is elevated. If it is due to a hypothyroid condition, then the best course of action is to treat the hypothyroid state. Statin drugs should only be used if the patient is suffering from statin-deficiency syndrome, and that just does not exist.

[1] Canaris, Gay, et al. The Colorado Thyroid Disease Prevalence Study. Arch. Intern. Med. Vol 160, Feb 28, 2000
[2] Harrison's Principles of Internal Medicine. 14th Edition. 1998
[3] Weetman, A.P. "Fortnightly review: Hypothyroidism: screening and subclinical disease." British Medical Journal. 1997;314:1175 919 April
[4] Hertoghe, Therese. From lecture at Broda O. Barnes M.D. Research Foundation, Stamford CT, February, 2002
[5] Barnes, Broda. IBID. p. 160-161

Chapter 13

Cholesterol and Iodine

CHAPTER 13: INTRODUCTION

The last chapter reviewed the relationship between hypothyroidism and heart disease. Recall that this relationship has been described in the medical literature for over 100 years. This chapter will expand on the relationship by discussing how iodine interacts with the thyroid gland and how iodine deficiency may be the underlying cause of most thyroid disorders as well as heart disease. I will show you why it is so important to ensure that you have adequate iodine intake. Low iodine intake can cause thyroid disorders, high cholesterol and heart disease.

THE HISTORY OF IODINE AND HEART DISEASE

In Western medicine, iodine was discovered in 1816 by an English physician, William Prout, who used it to treat a patient with goiter (swollen thyroid gland). The use of iodine in Western medicine could be considered to be the birth of Western medicine. In 1824, a French chemist, Boussingault, recommended the use of iodized salt to treat goiter. It was the first time a single substance—iodine—was recommended for a single condition. That is exactly how Western medicine is taught today. Medical students are taught to diagnose pathology then prescribe the drug to treat the malady.

Recall from Chapter 5, that the cholesterol = heart disease hypothesis started in the early twentieth century by a Russian researcher, Nikolai Anichkov. In 1913, he published his famous rabbit study where rabbits fed cholesterol developed atherosclerotic plaques in their aortas in a similar pattern to the way humans who have atherosclerosis do. The cholesterol = heart disease hypothesis train left the station after Dr. Anichkov's research was published.

However, what is not common knowledge is research showing that iodine supplementation could blunt the findings Anichkov reported.

RATS, IODINE, AND CHOLESTEROL

Five years after Anichkov's research was published, scientists demonstrated that feeding iodine to rabbits could prevent the deposition of cholesterol in the arteries of rabbits that were fed cholesterol. [1] Perhaps the cholesterol = heart disease hypothesis train should have been pulled over in 1918 and put to rest! However, Big Pharma had no desire to put that to rest, but I am getting sidetracked...

Interestingly, similar iodine and cholesterol studies were reproduced and similar results were reported in the literature four times.[2][3][4][5] One of those studies looked at rats fed an iodine-deficient diet versus rats fed an iodine-sufficient diet.[6] The iodine-deficient diet resulted in a four-fold higher thyroid weight as compared to the iodine-sufficient diet. When the rats were fed a high cholesterol diet, the thyroid weight significantly increased (indicative of goiter) in both groups. The high cholesterol diet was also found to increase the body's excretion of iodine.

This is an important study. It is easily predicted that the poor rats fed an iodine-deficient diet would suffer with goiter (a large thyroid gland) as iodine deficiency is well-known to cause thyroid problems including goiter.

What is much less known is the relationship between iodine and cholesterol. The rat study showed that a high cholesterol diet increased the body's need for iodine.

How does this rat study affect us? We live in a wealthy Western society. All wealthy Western societies eat a lot of cholesterol in their diets. If there is iodine deficiency present, eating a lot of cholesterol will worsen the iodine deficiency problem. This can lead to thyroid issues and heart disease.

IODINE, THYROID HORMONE, AND HEART DISEASE

Another study found that iodine deficiency in rats resulted in a subclinical hypothyroid picture—the poor rats had an elevated TSH with normal thyroid hormone levels which included both T4 and T3.[7] Recall from the previous chapter that T4 is the inactive form of thyroid hormone while T3 is the active form. Despite normal T3 levels, cardiac tissue was found to be deficient in T3. T4 therapy was unable to correct the cardiac deficiency, in the presence of iodine deficiency. T4 therapy refers to commonly used thyroid medications Synthroid® and Levothroid®. This study showed that iodine deficiency should be either corrected concurrently with the diagnosis of hypothyroidism or it should precede the treatment for hypothyroidism.

IODINE AND ITS RELATION TO CHOLESTEROL LEVELS

Researchers studied 136 subjects for their iodine intake and looked at their lipid parameters. Compared to iodine-sufficient, non-goiterous controls, iodine-deficient goiterous subjects had significantly higher average cholesterol levels and

LDL-cholesterol levels.[8]

It is interesting that the low-iodine group had higher cholesterol and LDL-cholesterol levels. This goes back to my earlier point that elevated cholesterol levels are a symptom of something wrong—like the warning lights in your car. In this case, the elevated cholesterol levels may be a signal that iodine levels are low.

I have treated thousands of patients with iodine. I have seen many improve their thyroid function with iodine therapy. Iodine may have a direct effect on cholesterol levels or it may improve the level by enhancing the functioning of the thyroid gland.

In 1958, Dr. Ancel Keys published data that countries with the highest cholesterol levels had the highest rate of cardiovascular disease.[9] At that time, in Europe, Finland had the highest rate of cardiovascular mortality, and it was more prevalent in Eastern versus Western Finland. Researchers looked at a variety of dietary components including:

- Amino Acids
- Carbohydrates
- Fats
- Lipids

- Minerals
- Proteins
- Vitamins

The researchers found the greatest statistical difference between Eastern and Western Finland was iodine intake. The risk of cardiovascular death was over 3.5x higher in individuals with goiter. And, there was a significantly lowered age of death in those with goiter.

In 1970, scientists looked at the prevalence of cardiovascular diseases in 21 Finnish cities as it related to trace elements in drinking water.[10] The trace elements studied included:

- Bromine
- Calcium
- Chlorine
- Fluorine
- Iodine

Cardiovascular endpoints were studied which included angina, coronary thrombosis, hypertension, and atherosclerosis. The strongest correlation with cardiovascular disease was iodine deficiency. The highest intake of iodine was associated with the lowest rate of cardiovascular disease.

Due to those studies, Finland increased iodine intake in its population by adding more to dairy feed and animal salt. The researchers concluded, "The author draws attention to other evidence that a low iodine intake may help to cause circulatory disease through an effect on thyroid metabolism and suggests that it might account for the high mortality rate from coronary heart disease in Finland…." In the past several decades, Finnish cardiovascular mortality has decreased by over 50% and life expectancy has increased by five years. Finland currently has the highest iodine intake of any European country. [11] [12]

IODINE, LIPIDS, AND INSULIN

Researchers studied 262 children living in an iodine-deficient area of Morocco. The subjects had an averaged TSH that was elevated. They were given a single 400mg oral iodized oil capsule. After six months, the researchers reported that the subjects had experienced a:

- Decrease in TSH
- Decrease in LDL/HDL

The authors reported, "Correction of iodine associated subclinical hypothyroidism improves the insulin and lipid profile and may…reduce the risk for cardiovascular disease."[13]   This is another study showing iodine improving lipid parameters.

Furthermore, this study found that iodine supplementation improved insulin levels.

Again, I will state that abnormal lipid levels are a signal that something is off in the body. It is not a signal for statin drugs.

There are a plethora of studies showing a relationship between low iodine levels and the development of hypothyroidism. I don't think anyone can say that iodine deficiency doesn't cause hypothyroidism.

IODINE DEFICIENCY OCCURRING AT EPIDEMIC RATES

Many physicians think that iodine deficiency is from the past. They will argue that iodized salt cured iodine deficiency. They are wrong.

I was taught in medical school that no one needed to supplement with iodine as iodine deficiency was not present in the U.S. It is amazing to me how incorrect statements keep getting repeated over and over.

Unfortunately, iodine deficiency is not only alive and well in our twenty-first century modern world but it is occurring at epidemic rates. Over the last 40 years, The U.S. National Health and Nutrition Examination Survey (NHANES) has found iodine levels have fallen over 50%s (see Figure 1).[14]

During the time iodine levels have fallen, we have seen epidemic increases of thyroid disorders—including hypothyroidism, autoimmune thyroid disorders and cancer—including cancer of the breasts, ovaries, uterus, pancreas, and prostate. All of the above conditions can be caused by iodine deficiency. In fact, it is my premise that we are seeing so many of the above conditions because of iodine deficiency. One of iodine's main jobs in the body is to maintain the normal architecture of the glands. The glandular tissue includes the thyroid, ovaries, uterus, breast, prostate, and pancreas.

FIGURE 1: NHANES IODINE LEVELS 1971-2012

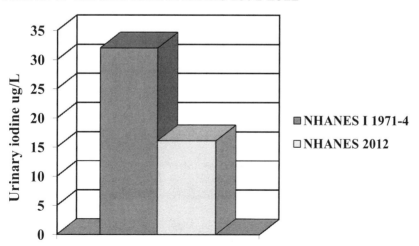

A further discussion of iodine's benefits is beyond the scope of this book. More information about iodine can be found in my book, *Iodine: Why You Need It, Why You Can't Live Without It.*

Final Thoughts

Iodine deficiency is occurring at epidemic rates. It is known to cause hypothyroidism. Medical literature is replete with articles dating back over 100 years correlating hypothyroidism with the development of heart disease.

I find it much more plausible that the epidemic of heart disease is caused (in part) by iodine deficiency rather than statin deficiency syndrome. Iodine deficiency can lead to a low thyroid condition—hypothyroidism.

Contrast the above statements with conventional medicine's approach of using statin drugs to prevent or treat heart disease. At best, the statin drugs lower one's risk for heart disease by 1-3.5%. However, the adverse effects alone negate that miniscule positive effect.

Finally, if heart disease is caused by a statin-deficiency syndrome, then I say take the statins. Otherwise it is best to search for an underlying cause of heart disease and treat that.

Iodine deficiency sounds more plausible than statin deficiency when talking about a potential cause of heart disease.

[1] Trans. Jpn. Path. 8:22104. 1918

[2] Arch. Exp. Pathol. Pharmokol. 159:265-274. 1931

[3] Z. Gesamte. Exp. Med. 87:683-702. 1933

[4] J. Exp. Med. 58:115-25. 1933

[5] Res. Commun. Chem. Pathol. Pharmacol. 1:169-84, 1970
[6] J. Exp.Med. 58. 1933. IBID
[7] J. Clin Invest. 1995;96(6):2828-2838
[8] Clin. Pediatr.208:123-8. 1996
[9] Lancet. 2:175-78. 1958
[10] Ann. Med. Exp. Et. Biol. Fenniae. 48: 117-121. 1970
[11] Prev. Med. 29:s124-9. 1999
[12] End. Exp. 20:35-47. 1986
[13] Thyroid. Vol. 19. 2009. DOI:10.1089/thy.2009.0001

14

Http://www.cdc.gov/nutritionreport/pdf/Nutrition_Book_complete508_final.pdf#zoom=100

Chapter 14

Diet and Heart Disease

CHAPTER 14: INTRODUCTION

For nearly 70 years, conventional medicine has searched for the reason why heart disease is our number one killer. During this time, The Powers-That-Be have assured us that they have uncovered the cause of heart disease: heart disease occurs because we eat too many saturated fats. The Powers-That-Be further state that eating too many saturated fats leads to elevated cholesterol levels. According to their theory, the elevated cholesterol levels are responsible for blocking the coronary arteries and causing heart disease. They further claim that if we lower our cholesterol levels, we will lower our rate of heart disease. However, there is very little data which shows that lowering cholesterol levels provides any measurable benefit in lowering the incidence of heart disease.

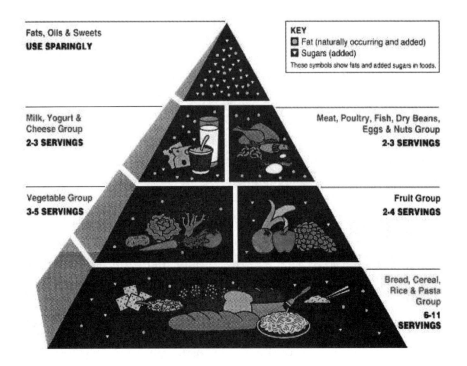

Figure 1: The Original USDA Food Pyramid

WHAT SHOULD WE EAT? THE FOOD PYRAMID

Nearly 25 years ago, the United States Department of Agriculture's (USDA's) food pyramid was designed to help Americans make better food choices so that they could overcome the epidemic of heart disease that was occurring. The original food pyramid is shown in Figure 1. You can see the USDA's food pyramid encourages the consumption of grain products and discourages the ingestion of fats and oils. Furthermore, the food pyramid told us to limit our intake of meat, eggs, and nuts. The

Powers-That-Be seized on this and the American Heart Association (a founding member of The Powers-That-Be) instructed all Americans to eat less saturated fat and consume more polyunsaturated fat in the form of vegetable oils.

In 1965, the American Heart Association (AHA) advised people to reduce cholesterol and fat in their diet with the idea that this would reduce their levels of serum cholesterol. According to The Powers-That-Be, reducing cholesterol levels would lower the risk for developing coronary heart disease. In 1977, U.S. public health dietary advice was announced by the Select Committee on Nutrition and Human needs.[1] The dietary recommendations focused on reducing dietary fat intake specifically to:

- Reduce overall fat consumption to 30% of total energy intake.
- Reduce saturated fat consumption to 10% of total energy intake.

In 2015, my THINCS colleague Zoe Harcombe, at the University of the West, Scotland, UK, and her team reviewed the data that was available to the scientists who wrote the 1977 guidelines. Harcombe found that there were no differences in all-cause or cardiovascular mortality in dietary groups that limited their fat intake. She found that the reductions in cholesterol were significantly higher in the intervention (low-fat diet) groups but this did not result in significant differences in coronary heart disease or all-cause mortality. This finding, alone, would negate the cholesterol = heart disease hypothesis. In fact, Harcombe found government dietary fat recommendations were untested in any trial prior to being introduced. She concluded, "Dietary recommendations were introduced for 220 million U.S. {citizens}...in the absence of supporting evidence from randomized controlled trials."

You might have to read those last two sentences again. The U.S. Government specified dietary guidelines without any evidence that it would actually work. I guess, by now, we should not be surprised. The consequence of lowering our fat intake has been severe; we have more obesity and diabetes than we know what to do with. Perhaps those that have been promoting the low-fat myth now have egg—with a large amount of cholesterol—on their face.

At the time the 1977 guidelines were trumpeted, there were other major studies that indicated that diet has little or no effect on serum (blood) cholesterol.[2][3] Remember, cholesterol is produced in the liver as well as by each and every one of the cells in the body. If you lower your dietary intake of cholesterol-containing foods, your body will adjust by producing more cholesterol. The inverse also holds true: if we eat more cholesterol, our bodies will produce less of it. In fact, according to Uffe Ravnskov, M.D., in his groundbreaking book *The Cholesterol Myths*, our bodies actually produce three to four times more cholesterol than our typical dietary intake of cholesterol.

So, what did we do with the recommendations from The Powers-That-Be? We were good citizens; we followed their advice. Over the years, we have consumed less total fat, including ingesting lowered amounts of saturated fat while increasing our consumption of polyunsaturated fat. What did that do to the rate of heart disease? Nothing. The rate of heart disease continued to rise even though Americans were lowering their intake of saturated fat and increasing their intake of polyunsaturated fat. The recent decline in mortality from heart disease does not correlate with the time period when we began to eat less saturated fats and more polyunsaturated fats. This decline began before Americans began lowering their fat intake.

At the same time we decreased our consumption of saturated fat, we also increased our intake of grains, primarily in the form of refined grains. In addition, we increased our intake of sugar. It is my premise that this increased intake of refined grains and sugar has been a double-whammy for us; it caused the epidemic of obesity and diabetes that we are currently facing.

Let me explain.

WE EAT TOO MANY REFINED GRAINS

Grains are a ubiquitous part of the human diet. They have been consumed by humans for a very short time period—relatively speaking–when you consider how long humans have inhabited this planet.

It is thought that humans evolved over a time period of approximately 1.5 million years. Throughout most of that time, humans survived by being hunter-gatherers; they ate what they could kill and pick. This included animal meats and organs, seafood, birds, insects, mushrooms, and fruits.

Approximately 11,500 years ago, humans began domesticating grains for consumption. Yes, there were some wild grains before then, but this is when the domestication of grains began. Corn was domesticated approximately 9,000 years ago but did not become a major staple in the diet until approximately 1,500 years ago.

Grains, like most plants, do not want to be eaten. Therefore, they produce toxins to discourage animals from eating them. Grains are high in phytic acid which is the principal storage form of phosphorus in many cereals and grains. In humans and other animals with a single stomach, the phosphorus is not available because it is bound to phytic acid. Phytic acid also binds to other plant-based minerals including calcium, magnesium, iron, and zinc which renders them non-absorbable to humans. Furthermore, phytic acid inhibits human digestive enzymes including pepsin, amylase, and trypsin which are needed to break down proteins and starch.[4]

Soaking, fermenting, and heating grains can disrupt phytic acid and allow humans to absorb the nutrients in grains. More about how to eat healthier can be found in my book, *"The Guide to Healthy Eating."*

The major problem with grains is that they turn into sugar very quickly in the body. Therefore, a diet high in grains could be expected to cause problems with elevated blood sugar. That is exactly what I see in my practice.

To be fair, eating unrefined grains is a better choice when compared to refined grains. Unrefined grains contain more vitamins, minerals, and enzymes as compared to refined grains. However, unrefined grains, like refined grains, similarly turn into sugar very quickly in the body.

My experience has clearly shown that a healthy diet minimizes the ingestion of grains, especially refined grains. For patients suffering with blood sugar issues, a grain-free (and sugar-free) diet has proven the best way to lower blood sugar, improve insulin sensitivity and lower markers of inflammation in the body such as cholesterol. Remember, cholesterol has strong anti-inflammatory capabilities and will increase when the body is suffering with excess inflammation. Since diabetes is a risk factor for heart disease, there is no better way to combat heart disease than to lessen the chance of getting as well as treating any existing diabetes.

ANDREA'S STORY

Andrea works in my office as the office manager. She is 61-years-old and in excellent health. Eight years ago, her internist prescribed Lipitor® to her during a routine doctor's visit. At that time, Andrea felt her health was excellent as she was feeling well. The doctor told her that she needed to take Lipitor® to prevent a heart attack due to her family history and because Andrea's cholesterol level was over 200mg/dl—it was 216mg/dl. Her physician told Andrea that her cholesterol was "well above normal".

By 2010, two years later, Andrea was not feeling well. "I could barely walk up the stairs in my home. I told my husband, 'We have to move to a one-floor house because I can't navigate the stairs'." At this time, Andrea also stated that her whole body ached. "This was very upsetting to me as I have worked out continuously for over 30 years. Before I started taking Lipitor®, I considered myself in great physical shape. After two years of taking Lipitor®, everything changed. I felt like I had turned into an old, crippled lady." At the office one day, Andrea came to me and told me what was going on. I told her that the aching muscles and generalized weakness were well-known adverse effects from taking statins. Andrea decided to stop taking Lipitor®. "I really had no choice as I was feeling so bad. After one month off the statin medication, I began to feel better. It was a slow process, but I began to resume my old exercise regimen and my muscles began to stop aching," she stated.

A year later, Andrea was feeling back to normal. However, her mother became very ill. Andrea was under a lot of stress and began to eat poorly. She was choosing comfort foods full of sugar and refined carbohydrates which are made from refined grain products. She went to her physician for a routine check-up and he again stated that her cholesterol level was too high. Andrea's blood test revealed:

- Cholesterol 268mg/dl
- LDL 178mg/dl
- Triglycerides 202mg/dl
- HDL 50mg/dl

Andrea's physician told her that her cholesterol levels were too high and that she would have a heart attack if she did not do something. He suggested that she try another statin medication. This time, Andrea asked for my opinion. I told her, "Do not take a statin medication as it has never been shown to prolong a woman's life or decrease her chance for a heart attack."

Andrea asked me if she needed to do anything about her cholesterol numbers. I asked her about her diet to which she told me she was eating too many comfort foods. "If you eliminate the whites—the refined sugar, flour, and salt-containing products, your cholesterol numbers will naturally come down," I stated. Furthermore, I told her that the elevated triglyceride level (>150mg/dl) was directly related to eating too much sugar and refined carbohydrates. Andrea said, "Well, I sort of eat like that already." I replied, "I didn't say 'sort of', I said 'eliminate'." I instructed Andrea to cut out all sugar as well as grains as they turn to sugar very quickly in the body. From that moment on, Andrea changed her diet, as instructed. Four months later, she had her blood drawn to recheck her cholesterol levels. Her new numbers revealed:

- Cholesterol 199mg/dl
- LDL 129mg/dl
- Triglycerides 133md/dl
- HDL 43mg/dl

When Andrea's internist saw the new cholesterol numbers he stated, "Your numbers look good, keep up the good work." More importantly to Andrea was that she felt well. Eating this way, she lost twenty pounds over six months and she experienced *no aching in her muscles and joints.*

I cannot understand why doctors are so quick to prescribe medications for lowering cholesterol while never counseling their patients about diet. In Andrea's case, her cholesterol numbers were indicating that something was wrong–she was eating a poor diet. I told Andrea to find a new internist. To this date, she is feeling well and still eats a diet free of refined carbohydrates and added sugars.

WHAT IS THE BEST DIET TO PREVENT OR TREAT HEART DISEASE?

After practicing medicine for over 20 years, I can assure you that there is not one perfect diet that works for everybody. Each human being is a unique biochemical individual that is best served by finding what works and does not work for him/herself.

One of the most frustrating parts of my practice is addressing a patient's diet. Those suffering with obesity and diabetes have been indoctrinated by The Powers-That-Be that eating a low-fat diet is healthy and contributes to weight loss. That simply is not true. We have become the most obese people on the face of the planet for two basic dietary reasons: We eat too many low-fat foods and we ingest too much sugar.

Low-fat food has been a disaster for America. Most low-fat food sources contain too much sugar and too many carbohydrates which quickly turn into sugar when digested. I always counsel my patients to avoid all low-fat food sources.

The human body needs and requires fat. As we followed the AHA and the USDAs recommendation to lower fat in our diet, we became heavier. Fat provides satiety while eating too many carbohydrates makes one hungrier. More information about fats can be found in my book, *The Skinny on Fats*.

Although delving into the intricacies of a heart-healthy diet is beyond the scope of this book, I would like to provide some general recommendations that can help you make better food choices.

FOUR BASIC DIETARY STEPS FOR OPTIMIZING HEALTH

In order to eat a healthy diet, there are four basic steps that anyone can adopt that will not only reduce your chance for developing heart disease, but also improve your overall health.

- **1. Avoid all refined foods**

As I previously mentioned, refined food sources are made from refined flour, salt, sugar, and oils. We ingest too much refined sugar, especially in the form of high-fructose corn syrup. All refined substances are devitalized food sources. They lack basic vitamins, minerals, and enzymes. Eating these items will lead to a devitalized body and promote illnesses such as heart disease. Choose unrefined sources of flour, salt, sugar, and oils.

- ## 2. Avoid Dehydration

One of the easiest things anyone can do to improve their health is to maintain hydration. What this means is to drink adequate amounts of water. How much water is this? Take your weight in pounds, divide by the number two and the resulting number is the amount of water in ounces you should ingest on a daily basis.

Water is the largest constituent of the human body—nearly 70% of the body and 80% of the brain is composed of water. Most of the new patients that I see are dehydrated—they simply do not drink enough water. A dehydrated state sets in motion a cascade of events that is detrimental to the body including elevating blood pressure and constricting of the arteries. Both of these factors can lead to heart attacks.

- ## 3. Maintain Adequate Salt Intake

Salt is the second major constituent in the body, next to water. We need adequate amounts of salt for maintaining cellular hydration and for proper adrenal function. Low salt levels can lead to an imbalanced adrenal hormone status. Studies have shown low-salt diets lead to elevated cholesterol, LDL-cholesterol, and insulin levels.[5][6] Perhaps The Big Pharma cartel, who profit from statin drugs, have a vested interest in promoting a low-salt diet.

In fact, a study of 3,000 hypertensive patients found a 430% (RR) increase in heart attacks in the group who ingested a low-salt diet compared to a group with the highest salt intake.[7] A study of 3,681 participants followed for nearly eight years found a significant, inverse correlation between low-salt intake and an increased risk of cardiovascular disease mortality.[8] In fact, this study found that the low-salt intake group, when compared to the high-salt intake group, had a five-fold increase in cardiovascular deaths. I know these studies seem counterintuitive since The-Powers-That-Be have continually lectured us that we need to lower our salt intake. They were and still are wrong. Salt is an essential substance for the human body. My testing has consistently shown that most patients (greater than 95%) are salt-deficient.

Could low-salt diets, as compared to higher-salt diets, actually cause more cardiovascular problems? Researchers have reported that, as compared with a high- salt diet, a low-salt diet has been associated with a greater than 400% (RR) increase in risk of myocardial infarction (heart attack) in men.[9] MRFIT (Multiple Risk Factor Intervention Trial), a study done by the National Heart, Lung and Blood Institute screened 361,662 men for a primary prevention trial looking at the effects of various interventions to lower mortality from heart disease. A very low-salt diet may provide minimal help lowering blood pressure in those that have hypertension. However, in people with normal blood pressure, there is little or no benefit from a blood pressure standpoint or a cardiovascular standpoint to justify instituting a low-salt diet.

Low-sodium diets predispose one to mineral and vitamin deficiencies including magnesium, potassium, and B-vitamins.[10] As previously stated, low-salt diets also promote elevated lipid and insulin levels. Each of these items could explain why a low-salt diet increases the cardiovascular risk.

What kind of salt should you ingest? Remember, I said to avoid refined salt. The healthiest salt is unrefined salt which contains over 80 essential minerals. Refined salt has no minerals. Two good forms of unrefined salt include Selina Naturally Celtic Sea Salt® and Redmond's Real Salt®. More information about salt can be found in my book, *Salt Your Way to Health*.

• 4. Eat Organic Food Free of Pesticides, Hormones and Antibiotics

Our food supply has become horribly adulterated. We ingest too many chemicals which disrupt the normal functioning of our bodies. Pesticides and antibiotics poison and alter the bacteria in our intestines. Synthetic hormones in our food supply disrupt our endocrine systems. All of these items promote inflammation which leads to elevated cholesterol levels. The best way to lower the inflammation levels in the body is to eat a healthier diet free of pesticides, hormones, and antibiotics.

FINAL THOUGHTS

Eating a healthy diet is one of the most important things you can do to prevent becoming a heart patient. Furthermore, eating a healthy diet is one of the most important things you can do to treat heart disease. The old adage "you are what you eat," is true.

The human body was designed beautifully. We are supposed to supply it with the raw materials it needs, including optimal amounts of protein, fat, and carbohydrates as well as vitamins, minerals, and enzymes. Eating a diet devoid of basic nutrients will cause problems in the body. The standard American diet (SAD), with its reliance on refined food sources, lacks basic nutrients. Eating SAD food products leads to a devitalized body and to the development of chronic illnesses such as heart disease.

Heart disease is an inflammatory illness. Lowering the levels of inflammation in the body is important for all cardiac patients and for those wishing to avoid becoming heart patients. The best way to accomplish this is to follow the steps I have outlined here and in my books.

More information about a healthy diet and about fat in the diet can be found in my books: *The Guide to Healthy Eating* and *The Skinny on Fats.*

[1] Select Committee on Nutrition and Human Needs. Dietary goals for the United States. 1st edn. Washington: US Govt Print Off, 1977
[2] Kannel, W.B. Kannel, W. B. and Gordon, T.: The Framingham Study. Diet and Regulation of Serum Cholesterol, Section 24, Dept. of Health, Education and Welfare, Washington, D. C., 1971
[3] Am. J. Clin. Nutr. 29:1384-92, 1976
[4] J. of Agricult. And Food Chem. 30(4):799-80. 1982
[5] NEJM. August 14, 2014
[6] J. Int. Med. 1993;233
[7] Alderman. Hypertension. 1995;25
[8] JAMA. May 4, 2011. Vol. 305, No. 17. 1777-85
[9] Alderman, M. Low urinary sodium is associated with greater risk of myocardial infarction among treated hypertensive men. Hypertension. 1995. Jun;25(6):1144-52
[10] Ann. Intern. Med. 1983;98(part2)

Chapter 15

Final Thoughts

CHAPTER 15: FINAL THOUGHTS

What causes heart disease? Is it caused by a statin-deficiency syndrome? Hopefully by now, you will agree with me that it is not.

Doctors should search for the underlying cause of illness before instituting a treatment plan. If physicians did that, we would all be spending a lot less on health care and we would not have a need for statin drugs.

Nearly forty years ago, a physician wrote about his search for the underlying cause of heart disease. His name was Broda Barnes, M.D. In 1976, he wrote *Hypothyroidism: The Unsuspected Illness.* It was one of the first health books that I read and it had (and continues to have) a big impact on my medical practice.

In Dr. Barnes' chapter titled, "The Thyroid and Heart Attacks," he described how doctors were busy trying to find the culprit behind the epidemic of heart disease that was affecting the country (as well as the world). Dr. Barnes wrote,

"Investigations of medical mysteries can be very much like those in fictional murder mysteries. First, one character becomes suspect, then another, and another, and another. The web of circumstantial evidence may seem almost complete. The suspects may look very much like murderers. Yet, in the end, the real criminal turns out to be someone previously unsuspected.

"Of suspected culprits behind heart attacks, seemingly likely causes of the coronary artery disease that leads to the attacks, there has certainly been no shortage. They have been highly publicized; you are undoubtedly aware of them and, quite likely, worried about them. But do they solve the mystery? Do they even begin to tell the story?"

Dr. Barnes' description of finding the culprit behind heart disease was prescient when he wrote it. Here we are, nearly forty years later, and we are still trying to solve the mystery. Over the last 70 years, conventional medicine has been focused on blaming cholesterol and dietary fat for causing heart disease even though the data clearly shows this is not the case. Unfortunately, we now have a plethora of toxic medications–statins–that lower cholesterol levels yet fail to significantly lower the risk of developing heart disease.

We need a new model. We spend too much on our health care, due in large part, to our overuse of expensive drugs that do not treat the underlying cause of illness. This book was written to help you make an informed choice about whether a statin medication is appropriate.

THE CAUSES OF HEART DISEASE

Until The Powers-That-Be understand the underlying cause(s) of heart disease, we will continue to waste untold amounts of health care dollars on medications that don't significantly alter the course of the illness and are associated with a plethora of serious adverse effects.

I have spent much of this book telling you why statin drugs do not work and why you should avoid them. That was the purpose of writing this book. However, I would also like to mention what I think are the underlying causes of heart disease and what you can do about them. Keep in mind that there is no single underlying cause of heart disease for every heart patient. We are each unique biochemical individuals with our own strengths and weaknesses. Conventional medicine needs to acknowledge that fact. Once it does, each patient can now be treated with an individualized regimen based on their particular condition.

INFLAMMATION AND HEART DISEASE

There is no question in my mind that inflammation is underlying all chronic and acute illnesses, including heart disease.

The statinophiles seize on this fact by pointing out that statin drugs have "pleiotropic" anti-inflammatory effects. They do. However, you cannot cure heart disease by taking an anti-inflammatory medication like a non-steroidal anti-inflammatory drug (NSAID) or a steroid. In fact, the long-term use of NSAIDS or steroids increase the risk of heart disease. Furthermore, statins are associated with other "pleiotropic" effects including myopathy, brain fog, and amnesia. More about the adverse effects of statins can be found in Chapter 9.

To understand the underlying cause of heart disease and any other illness fueled by inflammation, one must ask the question, "What is causing the inflammation?" I know it is a simple question, but the answer is not so simple. There are many factors that can cause inflammation and, secondarily, heart disease. I will provide you with a list of eight factors that I have found to cause heart disease. Each of these items causes inflammation in the body and subsequently increases the risk for developing heart disease.

1. CIGARETTE SMOKING

There is no question that cigarette smoking leads to an increase in inflammatory biomarkers. People who smoke cigarettes are two to four times more likely to get heart disease.[1]

Cigarette smoking can lead to an increase in oxidative stress on the lungs and the heart. Smoking reduces how much oxygen gets to the heart, raises the blood pressure, elevates the heart rate, and harms the lining of the blood vessels which can directly lead to heart disease. No one should smoke cigarettes.

2. INFECTIONS

There are many research studies correlating infections with the development of heart disease. In fact, the microbial hypothesis for an infectious agent causing heart disease has been described for over a hundred years. We know that infections are associated with an increase in death from cardiovascular disease.[2] [3] Bacterium such as mycoplasma and Chlamydial pneumonia and viruses such as Cytomegalovirus are known to cause and have been found in atherosclerotic lesions.[4] [5]

In Chapter 3, I showed you the data that LDL has important antibacterial effects. The worst thing to do in an infectious case is to give someone a medication, like a statin drug, that lowers LDL levels.

All heart patients should be tested and treated for underlying infections. I wrote about how underlying infections can cause autoimmune disorders in my book, *Overcoming Arthritis*.

3. HORMONAL IMBALANCES

In Chapter 11, I reviewed the adrenal and sex hormone biosynthetic pathways and showed you that statin drugs are bound to cause deficiencies of these hormones. There is a plethora of research showing that low testosterone levels are associated with the development and progression of heart disease. I have treated hundreds of cardiac patients, like I did with my father, who have significantly improved their condition once their hormonal system was restored to a healthy state. Other hormonal imbalances like DHEA and pregnenolone also contribute to heart disease.

Every heart patient should have a complete workup of his/her hormonal system. In fact, every patient who is trying to optimize his/her health should have a complete hormonal and nutritional evaluation.

4. HYPOTHYROIDISM

Chapter 12 discussed the connection between hypothyroidism and heart disease. It is well-established that a low thyroid condition can cause elevated cholesterol and inflammatory levels. Furthermore, for over 100 years, it has been known that hypothyroidism can cause atherosclerotic coronary heart disease. Every heart patient should have a full work up of his/her hormonal system including the adrenal and sex hormones as well as the thyroid gland.

5. NUTRIENT DEFICIENCIES

There are many research articles correlating low nutrient levels with the development of heart disease in both animals and humans. Studies have clearly shown that nutrient deficiencies such as B-vitamins as well as vitamins A, C, D, E, and K can all lead to heart disease. Beriberi or thiamine deficiency leads to heart disease.[6] Vitamin C deficiency can lead to scurvy and the subsequent development of heart disease. In fact, vitamin C deficiency has been shown to cause elevated cholesterol levels and elevated inflammatory markers associated with an increased heart disease risk.

Homocysteine is a protein produced in the body. It is directly related to B-vitamin levels, particularly vitamins B6 and B12 as well as folic acid. Elevated homocysteine levels have been correlated with the development of heart disease by oxidizing LDL particles.[7]

Some think that nutritional deficiencies are a thing of the past. I can guarantee you, that after checking thousands of patients for their nutritional status, that statement is false. The National Health and Nutritional Examination Survey (NHANES) continually finds that the vast majority of Americans are suffering from a variety of nutritional imbalances.

Every heart patient and every patient suffering from any chronic illness should have a complete nutritional evaluation to ascertain his/her vitamin and mineral levels.

6. Eating a Poor Diet

There is no doubt that we are suffering from so many nutritional deficiencies because, in large part, most Americans eat a poor diet. I reviewed the relationship between diet and the development of heart disease in Chapter 14. It is important to avoid refined food sources and eat whole food sources with a full complement of vitamins, minerals, and enzymes.

7. Dehydration

Dehydration can cause heart disease. It leads to thickened blood which can damage the arterial lining. Furthermore, it can lead to clots. Dehydration can also lead to electrolyte imbalances which can cause heart attacks. It is important to maintain optimal hydration—in fact it is the single most important thing you can do for your health.

I find the vast majority of my patients exhibit the signs of dehydration on a physical exam. Simply put, too many patients are not drinking enough water and, instead, are ingesting too many sodas and coffee drinks that pull water out of the body.

How much water should you ingest? Simply take your weight in pounds, divide the number by two and the resulting number is the amount of water you should ingest in ounces per day.

8. Heavy Metal Toxicity

I have checked thousands of patients for their heavy metal status. Unfortunately, my research has shown that the vast majority, over 80%, suffer from heavy metal toxicity. The two most common heavy metals found in my patients are lead and mercury. Elevated mercury levels have been shown to increase the risk of heart disease.[8] However, I have also found a significant number of my patients suffer from elevated levels of cadmium and nickel. All heavy metals cause an increase in inflammatory biomarkers. NHANES has found an association between heavy metal toxicities and heart disease.[9]

To minimize heavy metal exposure, avoid high mercury-laden fish such as tuna, swordfish and sea bass. Also, you should never let a dentist put a mercury amalgam filling in any living being's mouth. If your dentist still uses mercury fillings, I suggest that is a sign that you need to find a new dentist. They should know better.

Since most of us are loaded with toxic heavy metals, it is important to have your levels assessed and to undergo chelation if you have high heavy metal levels. Since no conventional physician is properly trained to do this, it is best to seek a holistic physician who is skilled in this technique. Appendix A will provide you with the information to find a holistic physician.

FINAL THOUGHTS

Until The Powers-That-Be admit that their model of what is causing heart disease is wrong, I see no real progress and no real solutions to combating the epidemic. It is important to reiterate the fact that heart disease is not the number one killer because we are suffering from an epidemic of statin-deficiency syndrome. This book should make it clear that statins are not the answer to reversing the epidemic of heart disease.

It is time for each of us to take control of our health care decisions. It is time for physicians to stand up and acknowledge that our drug-based model has failed. We are spending too much money on ineffective therapies. We must not rely on toxic medications that fail to treat the underlying cause of the heart disease epidemic. A holistic approach, which searches for the underlying cause and treats the cause, is a better model.

To All Our Health!

[1]

[2] Eur. Heart j. 1993. Suppl K:66-71
[3] Eur. H. J. 1993. SupplK:30-38
[4] The Lancet. Vol. 332. No. 8618. Octo, 1988. P. 983-986
[5] Circulation. 113:929-937. 2006
[6] Circulation. Vol VIII. November, 1953
[7] Nutr. Metab. Cardiovas. Dis. 1994:4:70-77
[8] NEJM. 347;1747-1754. 2002
[9] Angiology. Jul;62(5):422-9. 2011

APPENDIX: RESOURCES

1. To find a holistic health care provider, please contact The International College for Integrative Medicine (ICIM) at: www.icimed.com.

2. A compounding pharmacist can make a great part of your health care team. They can manufacture bioidentical hormones. To find a compounding pharmacist, please contact:

   The International Academy of Compounding Pharmacists (IACP) at: http://www.iacprx.org

   Phone: (800)-927-4227

   Fax: 281-495-0602

3. The International Network of Cholesterol Skeptics (THINCS). The International Network of Cholesterol Skeptics (THINCS) is a steadily growing group of scientists, physicians, other academicians and science writers from various countries. Members of this group represent different views about the causation of atherosclerosis and cardiovascular disease. More information can be found at: www.thincs.org.

4. Total Liver Care (TLC) can be ordered from Dr. Brownstein's office—The Center for Holistic Medicine—866.877.6467 or centerforholisticmedicine.com.

Index

A

Absolute Risk (AR) 106, 108-128, 198

Adverse drug reactions 157-190

ALS 163, 177, 179-181

Amnesia 172-176

Arsenic 211

ASCOT 111-118, 126-127, 137, 197

ATP 91, 93, 165

Autoimmune illness 163

B

Beta carotene 94

Bile 60, 94

Birth control pills 222

Blood clots 161

Breast cancer 163, 185, 194, 200-201, 221-222

Bromine 254

C

Cadmium 211

Cancer 163, 184-185, 199-201

Cataracts 163

Cholesterol Treatment Trialists' (CTT) 144-146

Chylomicrons 36

Congestive heart failure 167-169

CoQ10 92, 94-95, 163-169

Cortisol 208

Crestor 23, 120-124

D

Dementia 163, 172

Depo-Provera 161

Depression 163, 172, 231

DHEA 58, 208, 210, 217-219

Diabetes 149-150, 163, 183, 199, 215, 266

Dolichols 94, 96-97

E

Endotoxins 39-41

Estrogen 58, 208, 222-224

F

Fluorine 254

G

Gall bladder disease 214

Glutamate 180

Guillain-Barre syndrome 163, 177

H

HDL 33, 36-38, 42-45, 170, 214, 255, 272

HMG-CoA reductase 19, 90, 92, 94-95, 169

Hemochromatosis 242

Hypoadrenal 58

Hypogonadal 58

Hypothyroidism 18, 229-244

I

Insulin 255

Iodine 242, 249-259

Iron 269

Isoprenoids 94-96

J

JUPITER 118-124, 126, 197

K

Keys, Ancel 73-77

Kidney damage 163

Krebs cycle 93

L

LDL 33, 36-48, 136, 144, 147-149, 179, 182, 214, 255, 272

Lead 211

Lipitor 23, 112-115, 117-118, 128

M

Mercury 211

Mevalonate 90, 94-95

MSG 180

Multiple sclerosis 59, 177

Myalgia 163-164

Myelin 59, 176-179

Myopathy 163

Myositis 163

N

Neuropathy 163, 176, 178

Nickel 211

Number needed to treat (NNT) 107-108, 118, 139

O

Osteoporosis 161

P

Pancreatic cancer 185

Parkinson's disease 181-182

PCSK9 41, 45

Pregnenolone 58, 208, 210, 219-220

Progesterone 58, 161, 208, 210, 220-222

Proton pump inhibitors 90

Pulmonary edema 161

R

Ravnskov, Uffe 20, 58, 76

Relative risk (RR) 106, 109-128, 182, 198

Rhabdomyolysis 169-170

S

Salt 275-277

Serotonin receptor depletion 163

Sexual dysfunction 163

Skin cancer 163, 185

T

Testosterone 58, 208-210, 213-217, 220

Thyroid hormone 209, 213

Thyroxine (T4) 232-234, 252

Total Liver Care (TLC) 212

Transient global amnesia 173-176

Triglycerides 36-37, 40-41, 272

Triiodothyronine (T3) 232-234, 252

TSH 233-237, 252, 255

V

Vitamin A 94, 242

Vitamin B-2 165

Vitamin B-3 165

Vitamin B12 165

Vitamin C 165

Vitamin E 94, 165-166

Vitamin K1 94

Z

Zinc 269

Books by David Brownstein, M.D.
More information: www.drbrownstein.com

The Statin Disaster

Statin drugs are the most profitable drugs in the history of Big Pharma. The best of the studies show statin drugs fail to significantly lower your risk of developing heart disease. This book will tell you the truth about statin drugs. Statins are associated with a host of adverse effects including:

- ALS
- Breast Cancer
- Congestive Heart Failure
- Memory Loss
- *Myopathy*
- *Neuropathy*
- *Sexual Dysfunction*
- *Skin Cancer*

Vitamin B12 for Health

Vitamin B12 deficiency is occurring in epidemic numbers. This book show you the many benefits of using natural, bioidentical forms of vitamin B12 and how B12 supplements can help you achieve your optimal health. B12 therapy can treat many common ailments including:

- Anemia
- Autoimmune Illness
- Blood Clots
- Brain Fog
- Cognitive Decline
- Depression
- Fatigue
- Fibromyalgia
- Heart Disease
- Muscle Disease
- Neurologic Problems
- Osteoporosis
- AND MUCH MORE!

IODINE: WHY YOU NEED IT, WHY YOU CAN'T LIVE WITHOUT IT, 5th EDITION

Iodine is the most misunderstood nutrient. Dr. Brownstein shows you the benefit of supplementing with iodine. Iodine deficiency is rampant. It is a world-wide problem and is at near epidemic levels in the United States. Most people wrongly assume that you get enough iodine from iodized salt. Dr. Brownstein convincingly shows you why it is vitally important to get your iodine levels measured. He shows you how iodine deficiency is related to:

- Breast cancer
- Hypothyroidism and Graves' disease
- Autoimmune illnesses
- Chronic Fatigue and Fibromyalgia
- Cancer of the prostate, ovaries, and much more!

OVERCOMING ARTHRITIS

Dr. Brownstein shows you how a holistic approach can help you overcome arthritis, fibromyalgia, chronic fatigue syndrome, and other conditions. This approach encompasses the use of:

- Allergy elimination
- Detoxification
- Diet
- Natural, bioidentical hormones
- Vitamins and minerals
- Water

DRUGS THAT DON'T WORK and NATURAL THERAPIES THAT DO, 2nd Edition

Dr. Brownstein's newest book will show you why the most commonly prescribed drugs may not be your best choice. Dr. Brownstein shows why drugs have so many adverse effects. The following conditions are covered in this book: high cholesterol levels, depression, GERD and reflux esophagitis, osteoporosis, inflammation, and hormone imbalances. He also gives examples of natural substances that can help the body heal.

See why the following drugs need to be avoided:

- Cholesterol-lowering drugs (statins such as Lipitor, Zocor, Mevacor, and Crestor and Zetia)
- Antidepressant drugs (SSRI's such as Prozac, Zoloft, Celexa, Paxil)
- Antacid drugs (H-2 blockers and PPI's such as Nexium, Prilosec, and Zantac)
- Osteoporosis drugs (Bisphosphonates such as Fosomax and Actonel, Zometa, and Boniva)
- Diabetes drugs (Metformin, Avandia, Glucotrol, etc.)
- Anti-inflammatory drugs (Celebrex, Vioxx, Motrin, Naprosyn, etc)
- Synthetic Hormones (Provera and Estrogen)

SALT YOUR WAY TO HEALTH , 2nd Edition

Dr. Brownstein dispels many of the myths of salt—salt is bad for you, salt causes hypertension. These are just a few of the myths Dr. Brownstein tackles in this book. He shows you how the right kind of salt--unrefined salt--can have a remarkable health benefit to the body. Refined salt is a toxic, devitalized substance for the body. Unrefined salt is a necessary ingredient for achieving your optimal health. See how adding unrefined salt to your diet can help you:

- Maintain a normal blood pressure
- Balance your hormones
- Optimize your immune system
- Lower your risk for heart disease
- Overcome chronic illness

THE MIRACLE OF NATURAL HORMONES, 3rd EDITION

Optimal health cannot be achieved with an imbalanced hormonal system. Dr. Brownstein's research on bioidentical hormones provides the reader with a plethora of information on the benefits of balancing the hormonal system with bioidentical, natural hormones. This book is in its third edition. This book gives actual case studies of the benefits of natural hormones.

See how balancing the hormonal system can help:
- Arthritis and autoimmune disorders
- Chronic fatigue syndrome and fibromyalgia
- Heart disease
- Hypothyroidism
- Menopausal symptoms
- And much more!

OVERCOMING THYROID DISORDERS, 3rd Edition

This book provides new insight into why thyroid disorders are frequently undiagnosed and how best to treat them. The holistic treatment plan outlined in this book will show you how safe and natural remedies can help improve your thyroid function and help you achieve your optimal health. NEW SECOND EDITION!

- Detoxification
- Diet
- Graves'
- Hashimoto's Disease
- Hypothyroidism
- And Much More!!

THE GUIDE TO HEALTHY EATING, 2nd Edition

Which food do you buy? Where to shop? How do you prepare food? This book will answer all of these questions and much more. Dr. Brownstein co-wrote this book with his nutritionist, Sheryl Shenefelt, C.N. Eating the healthiest way is the most important thing you can do. This book contains recipes and information on how best to feed your family. See how eating a healthier diet can help you:

- Avoid chronic illness
- Enhance your immune system
- Improve your family's nutrition

THE GUIDE TO A GLUTEN-FREE DIET, 2nd Edition

What would you say if 16% of the population (1/6) had a serious, life-threatening illness that was being diagnosed correctly only 3% of the time? Gluten-sensitivity is the most frequently missed diagnosis in the U.S. This book will show how you can incorporate a healthier lifestyle by becoming gluten-free.

- Why you should become gluten-free
- What illnesses are associated with gluten sensitivity
- How to shop and cook gluten-free
- Where to find gluten-free resources

THE GUIDE TO A DAIRY-FREE DIET

This book will show you why dairy is not a healthy food. Dr. Brownstein and Sheryl Shenefelt, C.N., will provide you the information you need to become dairy free. This book will dispel the myth that dairy from pasteurized milk is a healthy food choice. In fact, it is a devitalized food source which needs to be avoided.

Read this book to see why common dairy foods including milk cause:

- Osteoporosis
- Diabetes
- Allergies
- Asthma
- A Poor Immune System

THE SOY DECEPTION

This book will dispel the myth that soy is a healthy food. Soy ingestion can cause a myriad of severe health issues. More information can be found online at: www.thesoydeception.com. Read this book to see why soy can cause:

- Allergies
- Cancer
- Osteoporosis
- Thyroid Disorders
- A Poor Immune System
- And, Much More!

The Skinny on Fats

The Skinny on Fat was written to educate you about the importance of consuming good sources of dietary fat. This book will teach you why we need fat and why we can't live without it. Good sources of dietary fat can:

- Prevent heart disease
- Promote weight loss
- Improve the immune system
- Help prevent chronic illness

DVD's of Dr. Brownstein's Latest Lectures Now Available!

DVD: Iodine–The Most Misunderstood Nutrient

DVD: The Statin Disaster

DVD: Overcoming Thyroid Disorders

DVD: Drugs That Don't Work and Natural Therapies That Do

DVD: Holistic Medicine for the 21st Century

DVD: Salt Your Way to Health

DVD: The Miracle of Natural Hormones

DVD: The Soy Deception

DVD: The Guide to a Gluten-Free Diet

DVD: The Guide to Healthy Eating

For More Information, Please Go To:
www.drbrownstein.com

Call 1-888-647-5616 or
send a check or money order

BOOKS $18 each!

Sales Tax: For Michigan residents, please add $1.08 per book.

Shipping : 1-3 Books: $5.00
4-6 Books: $4.00
7-9 Books: $3.00

Order 10 or more books: FREE SHIPPING!

VOLUME DISCOUNTS AVAILABLE. CALL 1-888-647-5616 FOR MORE INFORMATION

DVD's of Dr. Brownstein's Lectures Available! DVD's: $25.00 each

INFORMATION OR ORDER ON-LINE AT:
WWW.DRBROWNSTEIN.COM

You can send a check to: Medical Alternatives Press
4173 Fieldbrook
West Bloomfield, MI 48323